Praise for *Protect Your Energy*

"This book is a balm to my nervous system. Zabie Yamasaki does so much more than remind us to rest—she helps us lay the groundwork for a life that feels nourishing and supportive, even in challenging times."

ALEX ELLE
author of *After the Rain* and *How We Heal*

"In this beautiful ode to lightening our loads, Zabie Yamasaki shows us the true strength in living more softly. With nervous-system-informed practices, these teachings don't just shape our calendars but help our bodies and minds find more ease in the busyness of life. A must-read for these times."

EVE RODSKY
author of *Fair Play* and *Find Your Unicorn Space*

"*Protect Your Energy* is a balm for our times. With tenderness and clarity, Zabie offers not just permission but practical tools to reclaim our wholeness in a world that pulls us away from ourselves. Through lived wisdom, embodied science, and soulful practice, she guides us home to our bodies and reminds us that rest, boundaries, and self-tending are acts of liberation. This book is an invitation to soften, to breathe, and to remember that everything we need is already within us."

DEVI BROWN
well-being educator, host of *Deeply Well*, author of *Living in Wisdom*

"*Protect Your Energy* feels like sitting with a trusted friend, reminding you to slow down, breathe, and honor the sacred within you. A timely guide for our times."

LALAH DELIA
author of *Vibrate Higher Daily*

"*Protect Your Energy* gently guides readers through deeply nourishing practices, reflections, and teachings that will liberate the heart, mind, body, and spirit of all who read it. Zabie's uniquely compassionate, wise, and tender words are like medicine in this fast, often over-whelming world. This book offers a source of heart-full support, expansive expertise, and embodied care for all who are longing for more ease, peace, and presence. What a true gift."

LISA OLIVERA
LMFT, author of *Already Enough* and *When the Ache Remains*

"Zabie Yamasaki has curated a permission slip in book form. These words are a necessary soft landing for the overachiever readers of the room who often confuse the emotions and fears of others as their own. This book could not have come at a better time for those of us who are overwhelmed, overstimulated, and looking to invite more ease into their lives. May this book be your guide."

ARIELLE ESTORIA
poet, actor, speaker, author of *The Unfolding*

"Zabie's work is transcendent and vital. Her book is not just an incredible guide to calm, but it's also a rallying cry not to do more, but to do less. Zabie's voice is a breath of fresh air!"

JAMIE VARON
author of *Radically Content*

"With wisdom, clarity, and tenderness, Zabie Yamasaki shares the healing gift of authentic guidance for our overscheduled, overstimulated, and often disconnected lives. If you are feeling exhausted, stressed, numb, or overwhelmed, this book offers a clear and loving perspective on how to nourish and care for yourself with sustainable and accessible practices. Couched in an understanding and deep respect for each individual's nervous system, this transformative book invites readers to feel into what is best for them personally. Throughout the book, Zabie gently invites readers to meet themselves where they are and embrace themselves with acceptance, love, and care. I highly recommend this book—a much-needed refuge for our times."

WENDY O'LEARY
public speaker, co-author of *Growing Self-Compassionate Children*, author of *It's OK*

"What compassionate wisdom for somatic resilience! With her background as a trauma-informed yoga educator, Zabie brings undeniable authority and unwavering empathy. The book is a collection of approachable, body-centered practices paired with supremely kind language. You come away feeling both seen and empowered. Zabie helps us out with this somatic toolkit based in healing for real life."

SUSANNA BARKATAKI
author of *Ignite Your Yoga* and *Embrace Yoga's Roots*

"As a trauma therapist, I've read countless resources on trauma-informed care, but this one truly resonates. In a world that constantly pulls us away from our center, Zabie's words offer a sacred and tender landing space for our nervous system. With grace and depth, she weaves her lived experience, clinical wisdom, and an extraordinary gift for language that both holds and heals. This resource is a gift, full of practical yet powerful practices to navigate protecting your precious energy. An essential companion for both personal reflection and professional practice."

CHRISTINE MARK-GRIFFIN, LCSW, RYT, EMDR
consultant, author of *EMDR Workbook for Kids*

"Reading *Protect Your Energy* feels like being wrapped in a warm weighted blanket. On every page, Zabie's soothing voice offers wisdom and compassion. She seamlessly weaves together her expertise on burnout and nervous system repair, along with the depth of her own lived experience. Zabie's eloquent words, along with the poignant quotes she curates, will stay with you long after you finish her book."

MOLLY NOURMAND, LMFT
founder and clinical director of Life After Birth®

"As a therapist, I've read countless books that promise restoration but few that deliver it the way *Protect Your Energy* does. Zabie Yamasaki writes with the rare combination of clinical wisdom, lived experience, and deep humanity. Every page is infused with her heart-centered approach—an invitation not only to soothe the individual nervous system but to imagine what collective, systemic healing could look like if rest and compassion were at its core.

This isn't a book about quick fixes or self-optimization. It's a reclamation. It is remembering that tending to our own energy is an act of resistance in a culture that profits from our exhaustion. Zabie's voice is both balm and blueprint: gentle, grounded, and profoundly transformative.

Protect Your Energy will become a companion for anyone who has ever over-given, over-functioned, or quietly burned out while caring for others. I'll be recommending it to my clients, my colleagues, and every healer I know. *Protect Your Energy* is a meditation in tending to ourselves in a world that encourages and rewards functioning from a place of over-productivity. This book changed my life."

SAHAR MARTINEZ, PSY.D, LMFT, PMH-C
founder, The Process Wellness Collective

"*Protect Your Energy* is the book I have been longing for—for myself and for those I love—as we try not just to survive but truly thrive amidst the heartbreaks of our world. It invites us into a slower, softer, and simpler way of being so we can listen to our deepest needs and honor them without apology. Zabie helps us to know that relief is possible and living with ease is within our power."

EILEEN S. ROSETE
author of *To Tend and To Hold*

protect your energy

Also by Zahabiyah A. Yamasaki

Trauma-Informed Yoga for Survivors of Sexual Assault: Practices for Healing and Teaching with Compassion

Trauma-Informed Yoga Affirmation Card Deck

Trauma-Informed Yoga Flip Chart: A Teaching Tool for Healing Professionals

Your Joy Is Beautiful: The Magic of Remembering That You Are Enough, Just as You Are

H Is for Healing Card Deck: 52 Everyday Practices to Strengthen Children's Emotional, Physical, and Mental Well-Being

protect your energy

A Gentle Guide to Nurture Your Nervous System, Cultivate Rest, and Honor Your Needs

Zahabiyah A. Yamasaki
MEd, RYT

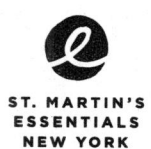

ST. MARTIN'S
ESSENTIALS
NEW YORK

First published in the United States by St. Martin's Essentials, an imprint of St. Martin's Publishing Group

EU Representative: Macmillan Publishers Ireland Ltd, 1st Floor, The Liffey Trust Centre, 117–126 Sheriff Street Upper, Dublin 1, D01 YC43

This book is not intended as a substitute for the medical recommendations of physicians, mental health professionals, or other health-care providers. Rather, it is intended to offer information to help the reader cooperate with physicians, mental health professionals, and health-care providers in a mutual quest for optimal well-being. We advise readers to carefully review and understand the ideas presented and to seek the advice of a qualified professional before attempting to use them.

Cover design by Jess Morphew
Cover and book design by Charli Barns
Illustrations © 2026 by Maggie Locktenburg
www.stmartins.com

The Library of Congress Cataloging-in-Publication Data is available upon request.

ISBN 978-1-64963-322-4 (trade paperback)
ISBN 978-1-64963-323-1 (ebook)

Our books may be purchased in bulk for specialty retail/wholesale, literacy, corporate/premium, educational, and subscription box use. Please contact MacmillanSpecialMarkets@macmillan.com.

First Edition: 2026

10 9 8 7 6 5 4 3 2 1

Dearest G,

I will never forget when my sister said at our wedding, "Remember to take care of Garrett, as he always does of you, because while you're out there saving the world, there is someone at home saving you." Her words continue to be an anchor in every sense of the word.

Thank you for loving me the way that you do. For creating the space for me to do work that I love. For reminding me that I am worthy of the care and compassion I pour into others. For soothing my anxiety with hugs, weighted blankets, and lavender oil on my temples. For being my biggest fan. For helping me pick up the pieces and put them back together differently. You, my love, are magic, and I am in awe of you. I love the life we have created together through intention, unwavering support, strength, resilience, and mutual respect.

May the words in this book reflect all the ways we have nurtured each other and our precious Grayson, Hudson, and Leilani. I love you.

To all the sensitive souls on the journey to embracing their softness and reconnecting to the parts that have gotten lost in service to others.

In a world that glamorizes "big breakthroughs," the truth is that most of the healing work actually lies in the small, slow, tedious, digestible process of showing up for ourselves over and over and over again. Keep going.
—THAÍS SKY, MA, LMFT

I used to separate good days from bad until I thought of myself as an ocean. I used to split times I felt strong from when I felt weak until I imagined myself as the sea. Calm and rocky, wild and soft, still and powerful and vast and more than any one thing. In the ocean it's hard to divorce one mood from another, one wave from the next. Now, on my worst days, I think of how good life is too, how I still can greet joy while swimming through grief. How fragile strength feels. How I'm not any one thing in any one moment on any one day. I'm all of it and all of it is me.

—HANNAH ROSENBERG

Gentle Reminders

Doing less is medicine for your nervous system.

Slowing down is medicine for your nervous system.

Pacing yourself is medicine for your nervous system.

Integration is medicine for your nervous system.

Being gentle with yourself is medicine for your nervous system.

Honoring your changing capacity is medicine for your nervous system.

Tending to your needs is medicine for your nervous system.

Managing your energy instead of your time is medicine for your nervous system.

Self-compassion is medicine for your nervous system.

Rest is medicine for your nervous system.

Contents

Foreword

Tracee Stanley, author of *Radiant Rest*

My prayer for us all is that we learn the sacred tools of protection—not as a way of separation, but as a way of being together while remembering and safeguarding our wholeness. And by doing so, we each become more conscious and careful with how we use our words, our power, and our own energy. That we hold ourselves sacred, along with every other living being and the earth, and from that place of true wholeness, we collectively weave a blanket of protection that has room for everybody and cocoons the whole world.

During the pandemic of 2020, when the world stopped moving and we were in the midst of the global lockdown, many of my friends, students, and colleagues, faced with the reality of halting the fast pace of their lives for what they thought would be a short time, said with some relief, "Well, now I can finally get some rest." As a teacher of meditation, ritual, and yoga nidra, I began offering classes to my online community and friends. For many, the time away from a structured schedule, work, and other responsibilities revealed layers of profound exhaustion that had been lurking below the surface of constant doing and urgency that had permeated their lives.

Yet the deep desire and need for rest beyond sleep seemed to be met with an equal and opposite force to push, to keep going, to be productive—to resist the inner call to rest. I began to wonder what it is that makes us keep going when we know we need to rest. What keeps us from pressing pause even for a few minutes to anchor into the gift of breath and observe our inner landscape? What are we so exhausted from? What are we running from or toward?

To get to the root of our resistance, we may consider the following questions: Is it safe to rest? Why am I so exhausted? Many times, we may imagine that we can retreat to a peaceful place and rest, but that isn't always true. At other times, we may feel that there is no safe place.

Thanks to teachers like Zabie and others, we have learned that not every sacred space is a safe space for everyone. We have varied experiences and are each on our own timeline of healing. When I read Zabie's first book, *Trauma-Informed Yoga for Survivors of Sexual Assault*, in 2021, it came at the right time to answer some of these questions, and I added it to the required reading for my yoga nidra teacher trainings. Teachers need tools that build on the desire to create spaces where folks can honor where they are in their process, and that is a minute-to-minute, nonlinear journey. But it is not just teachers and healers that need these tools. And I have often considered that perhaps more than a "safe space," we need a protected space. Much of our exhaustion stems from the constant need to protect ourselves and not knowing how. In a world that is becoming increasingly polarized and unstable, practices of protection should be part of our daily energetic hygiene. When practiced with awareness, these exercises can become generative and nourishing rather than exhausting.

2020 may seem like a long time ago, but we are still in transitional times—a space where the chasm of the unknown appears more stretched out than usual. While it is true that we are always in a state of transition (every breath and every moment of the day contains within it the natural cycle of birth, death, and rebirth), something feels different. Perhaps it was the pandemic that heightened our awareness of transitional spaces and the need to protect our energy. I have felt it; maybe you have too. I am grateful to Zabie for bringing this work forward, once again, at a time when the need is so great.

Introduction

Sending love to all those who hold the default nervous system in the room, whether through parenting, caregiving, leadership, teaching, or your profession. You deserve spaces where you are held in care. You are worthy of support with the mental load you carry. You deserve to rest.

Welcome, beloved, to what I hope will feel like the softest and most affirming place to land. Before we begin this journey of energetic reclamation together, I invite you to take a deep inhale and a restorative exhale to the degree that feels available to you here. It might feel supportive for you to relax your shoulders up, back, and down. Explore what it's like to release all the weight and tension you are carrying, even if just for a moment, within the container of this space. Allow whatever you might be holding to gently cascade to the earth, and notice the support that holds you here.

If you would like, take a moment to compassionately rest a palm on your heart and rub your chest in a soothing circular motion. I invite you to turn the volume of your heart all the way up and the volume of your thoughts all the way down. Start to arrive here with the full senses of your mind, body, and spirit. Know that everything you are holding is valid and welcome in this space. You are celebrated. You are seen. You are cherished. You are not alone in all of the heaviness that can come with just human-ing our way through this life.

When survival mode has become your baseline, learning how to rest and nurture flexibility in your nervous system, like you just did here, is an everyday practice that requires gentleness, tenderness, and self-compassion. Throughout this book, I will challenge you to explore speaking a little kinder to the parts of you that need softening and care, and encourage you to commit to nurturing yourself and trusting in the embodied shifts that are taking place, even when it might be hard to notice. It may be difficult to offer yourself grace and compassion at first, but the positive results will speak for themselves.

> **One of the most beautiful things about who you are right now is all the versions of you that kept going so you could get here.**[1]
> —NAKEIA HOMER

In my own nonlinear healing journey, there were many times when I felt tired of waking up each day trying to operate and function from an empty well. I was tired of measuring my worth based on how productive I was. I was tired of trying to live my life by traditional means of "success" instead of leaning into the courage of redefining what success could look like. I was tired of my health being an afterthought and pushing through debilitating panic attacks. I was tired of unrealistic expectations from employers and working myself to pieces. I was tired of blaming myself instead of the systems, ignoring my sensitivity and associating it with stigma and shame, and struggling to be present with my loved ones. Even more importantly, I was tired of normalizing all of these things.

You might find yourself feeling the same right now mentally and emotionally, realizing that this way of living is only harming you and wanting to make a change. You may feel like this is the way life is supposed to be or that you are simply unable to keep up. But I assure you that this is not the case. The way we have been taught to live and perform in our modern society goes against our nature, and this is why it feels so difficult to keep up. This journey we will embark on together is not about a magic formula or a checklist of more things to do to improve your well-being. In this book, I want to help you focus on doing *less* to protect your energy, reclaim yourself and your time, honor your needs and sense of embodied boundaries, and savor all the sacred moments in between. You deserve to rest.

My Lens

For as long as I can remember, my wounds and gifts have been bound together. And if there is one thing that is true for me, it's that grief and joy are close companions. As someone who navigates the world with a highly sensitive nervous system, finding a road map to protecting my energy has taken time, patience, self-kindness, and more trial and error than I would like to admit. Learning the process of showing up for myself daily and celebrating the choices I have with my body, mind, and spirit have changed my life. With these choices comes the affirming reminder that recovering from burnout and overwhelm is not a linear journey, and leaning into gentleness is medicine when our spirits are recalibrating.

To give you some context, I am a mother, a South Asian woman, a daughter of immigrants, and a survivor of sexual assault. I have experienced the loss of my beloved child twenty-six weeks into my pregnancy, held space for my mother and husband through their unique cancer journeys, wrote my first book during a global pandemic while working full-time and caring for my two-year-old, overcame many seasons of rolling panic attacks, and navigated the toxicity and burnout of working in academia and student affairs. Through it all, life kept life-ing, which is why taking what felt like a "radical" approach (in reality, it was more like a human approach) was the path that always tugged on my heartstrings. Deep down in my heart, I knew there was another, more soul-nurturing way to exist.

In her book *Women, Culture & Politics*, Angela Davis—feminist, political activist, academic, and author widely known for her involvement in the Black liberation movement —reminds us that *radical* simply means "getting to the root."[2] I have never been a traditional "rule follower" or someone who has colored inside the lines. Perhaps my spirit has always been too expansive to be trapped by the traditional boxes our societal systems often try to keep us in. My journey has been about identifying the root of our chronic exhaustion and working toward cultivating an internal sense of ease that felt *overflowing* instead of choppy and fleeting. Can you relate to grasping for ease and simultaneously feeling it slip through your fingers?

I have been in a relationship with the word *ease* for several years. Ease is the intention I set nearly every time I step onto my yoga mat. Ease is what I always tell my therapist I need more of in my life. Ease is my anchor during moments of overwhelm or crisis. It may not always feel attainable, but there is a mutual reciprocity that staying in the overflow will gently reveal. Those moments typically arrive in seasons where I have given myself the gift of stillness instead of leaning into my tendency to overwork myself into exhaustion as a means of coping. Clarity and wisdom tend to surface when we give ourselves the gift of spaciousness, regulation, and rest. Have you ever wondered why some of your best ideas come to you while you are taking a bath, during your meditation practice, when you intentionally *slow* down, or simply when you have offered yourself grace?

Sometimes that peaceful place we cultivate feels fleeting because of the fear of what might happen next. Surviving trauma has also allowed me to view joy in ways I don't think I ever knew how to access. None of us are defined by the hard things we go through, but of course they inform and shape the way we move through the world, the triggers we navigate, who we feel safe with, and so many other emotionally charged experiences we hold and carry daily. In addition to all the hard things that have quite literally pushed me to my edges, there are things I have clung to that are so intertwined into who I am: my softness, my sensitivity, my tenderness. I didn't always know this, but now I view them as signs of strength.

The complexity of all that we can hold and feel as humans deeply moves me. For me, anchoring back into joy means leaning into the overwhelming love I have for my beautiful children and my beloved husband, cherishing and nurturing my support system of incredible family and friends who help me feel seen and bring my nervous system ease, and feeling pride in the successful trauma-informed consulting business that I birthed from my deepest wounds. On other days, joy is as simple as getting excited about the little things, like morning coffee, sunsets, ocean walks, a vase of fresh flowers, the softest sweatpants, a stack of books, and flowy dresses.

To know that we are never just one thing, one story, or one experience and that we get to honor and hold the multidimensional aspects of our lives is such a gift. We can acknowledge the trials that build us into who we are, but we can also hold space for the bounty of pleasures that carry us through. In case no one has told you lately: I am so in awe of you and how far you've come with everything you've been navigating. I am so sorry for how strong and resilient you've had to be all these years. I can imagine how tired and exhausted you are. I am holding the hope that the heaviness lifts soon. Through this book and our time together, may you start to feel the pockets of light and joy. You are seen through it all.

The Journey to Protect Your Energy

A trauma mindset will convince you that everything will collapse if you're still, if you rest, or if you do something just for you. It's not true. Let some ease into your day, into your breath, into your life.[3]
—DR. THEMA BRYANT

I'll never forget when my dear friend and colleague dr. shena young, a body-centered psychologist and healer, texted me this: "You don't have to just survive anymore. You can breathe and choose to live." Sometimes the right words in a single moment can rearrange your insides. Her words fundamentally shifted something within my physiology and offered me the awareness I needed to begin the journey of intentionally breaking out of survival mode. This was a place where I had set up camp for far too long.

Navigating the world from a consistent state of hyperarousal meant always feeling anxious, on edge, and stressed. The chaos was familiar, and I struggled to let ease in without bracing myself for the next shoe to drop. It was hard to believe that anything good in my life would last. But the thing about honoring our unique journey is that it can be slow and intentional. The "breakthroughs" don't have to happen overnight and with intensity. The small, daily choices and embodied shifts matter, and they accumulate in the most beautifully affirming ways. I don't think we can be reminded of this enough. Sometimes we put far too much pressure on ourselves to speed up our growth, but there are no rules for what it has to look like.

Growth can be slowness for the nervous system, releasing urgency and creating space. Growth can be letting ourselves fall apart without the pressure to quickly "fix" or "find a solution." The world offers us such little time to be untethered, to grieve, or to just be with our feelings as they are. I find myself constantly telling my son, "Sweetheart, your pace is perfect." And I honestly have to remember to say the same words to myself. My wish for all of us is to release and soften our grip as much as we can allow.

As I began my journey of living my life outside of the crushing expectations of others, I started to realize that peace had been quietly awaiting me on the other side. Like a warm, cozy blanket and the most delicious cup of coffee, it was ready to wrap me in the compassion and care I had been searching for, for years. This was a place I had been yearning for but didn't quite know how to reach. A place that felt so hard to obtain, but also necessary for my health and well-being. A place that was not a luxury or something I could buy (like the wellness industry wants us to believe) but was essential for the sustainability of my being and my life. It was my soft place to land, and I had to be in a place where I was ready to receive a more peaceful way of being, a less urgent lifestyle, and a commitment to what Nicola Jane Hobbs, a psychologist and the author of *The Relaxed Woman*, refers to as "an unhurried presence."[4]

I was comfortable pouring into others, but some of the most breathtaking moments of my healing journey came when I truly learned to pour into myself. And not just in the "Let me squeeze that yoga class in at the end of an exhausting day" type of pouring. These were the radical, everyday life choices and boundaries that centered my care and made me a higher priority on my to-do list. It was about giving myself permission to take up more space in my life. I knew my nervous system was slowly healing when I could rest unapologetically, when I didn't see everything as an emergency, when I stopped packing my schedule, and when I started to respect my time and energy.

Sometimes the revolution is quiet. Sometimes it is trusting your internal cadence. The rhythm of your heartbeat. It is honoring what arises in the quiet moments with yourself. It is bringing awareness and attention to the many parts of you that need tending and responding in ways that feel kind, compassionate, supportive, and aligned.

My Work in the World

As a trauma-informed yoga teacher and national trainer, a resilience and well-being educator, a keynote speaker, and the founder of Transcending Trauma through Yoga, my work has touched tens of thousands of people in ways that still move me beyond words. I had a humble beginning as a "traveling" yogi with ten yoga mats in the back of my car, driving from rape crisis centers to trauma agencies to universities to teach my eight-week trauma-informed yoga series for survivors. The energy of community and healing in each of these spaces was so deeply palpable. Folks could show up and feel seen and enough just as they were. They could be vulnerable, and they were reminded that they do not have to hold it all together. They could receive nourishment and support when they were overwhelmed. They could say no and honor their capacity without feeling judged. They could be reminded that just pausing and existing is enough. I can think of so few spaces in this life where we are invited not to rush, to exist slowly in this way.

I used to teach a weekly donation-based trauma-informed yoga-as-healing class that brought together veterans, folks navigating divorce, survivors of sexual assault and domestic violence, and those moving through their healing journey in the aftermath of multiple experiences of trauma. I also started sharing this trauma-informed yoga framework and philosophy, along with inspiration for gentler and softer ways to exist, on Instagram: @transcending_trauma_with_yoga. There is something incredibly moving about a community of humans coming together to heal without ever having to share any details about what they have experienced or endured. Just the gentle presence of energy, empathy, compassion, and understanding. Over thirteen years, I've been able to cultivate this beautiful community into one that now includes over fifty-five thousand humans who touch my heart daily with messages about how Transcending Trauma through Yoga has fundamentally changed their lives.

This work continued to unfold in magical ways, and I ultimately started to lead trauma-informed yoga certification trainings for healing professionals as well as provide consultations for universities and trauma agencies that are passionate about holistic frameworks of care and integrating trauma-informed yoga into their scope of services. When I first started this work, Stanford was one of the first universities to hire me. I literally could not believe they wanted my help in building an integrative model into their services for survivors.

After tending to the imposter syndrome, I looked myself in the mirror and felt that a big shift in my life and work was coming. The successful implementation at Stanford led to several other referrals, and before I knew it, we were implementing the trauma-informed yoga curriculum at over fifty universities and agencies, including the University of California system, the University of Southern California, Yale University, the University of Notre Dame, and Johns Hopkins University. I still remember the day CNN interviewed me for my work. I was two months postpartum, incredibly tender and emotional, and in awe of the way my dream had taken flight. I reflect on this journey often and hold it with so much gratitude. I say all of this to remind you that your dreams are worthy of tending to, and it's safe to follow your heart.

For as long as I can remember, I have let my sensitivity and softness guide my life and work. Many of us have internalized messages that our sensitivity is something we should hide or be ashamed of. But our sensitivity reveals the depth of our hearts and passions, and allows us to be more attuned and empathetic to the needs of others. **Staying soft in a hard world is something to be proud of. Your sensitivity is truly such a gift.**

My heart has been drawn to the courage, resilience, and strength that humans can access even amid the unfathomable. This energy and heart-centered space has fostered the most incredible career and brought a beautiful and inspiring community into my life. Over the years, my commitment to soulful activism and to the trauma-and nervous system–informed field of work has broadened its scope. It has reached an even wider audience of folks who can benefit from somatic tools and, most importantly, more gentleness and tenderness.

If you have journeyed with me for a while, you may know that my previous published work focused specifically on trauma and survivors. This new book draws upon trauma-informed concepts rooted in psychobiology to offer practices that help us face daily stressors, energy drains, and systemic injustices with more ease and capacity. In a world that puts so much pressure on humans to compartmentalize themselves, these pages offer an affirming road map to heal disconnection and disembodiment with the goal of self-integration and nervous system regulation, regardless of background or lived experience.

Why This Book

So many of us feel pressured to hold it all together, care for others, and survive in systems and frameworks that are not set up for us to thrive. There are so many systemic reasons why we carry the various burdens we do, including but not limited to racism, classism, ableism, ageism, gender inequality and oppression, LGBTQIA+ discrimination, and body-size discrimination. Systems of oppression are intersectional in nature and often embedded into society and governmental structures, which adds to the everyday exhaustion historically marginalized folks experience as they navigate the world. Whether you're experiencing a lack of affordable childcare and housing, medical or legal discrimination, or a lack of accessible mental health resources, please know you are not alone in your experience.

Additionally, at a psychobiological level, our nervous systems are constantly absorbing information through our environments, work, relationships, media, and even activism, which can leave embodied residual imprints and deplete the energy we bring into the world. As the podcast creator and author Kathryn Nicolai reminds us, in a single morning, we absorb more messaging, news, and images than our ancestors did in their entire lives.[5] Our nervous systems were not designed for this kind of lifestyle, but for many of us, this state of perpetual overwhelm, information overload, and exhaustion has become the norm. This has serious consequences for our mental, spiritual, emotional, and physical health.

In response, this book aims to serve as a restorative love letter of sorts; an antidote that offers a compassionate and gentle voice in a very loud and opinionated world. There is a sea of voices out there that may be pointing you to quick fixes, trends, and *more* of everything. **But the truth is sometimes what our nervous systems actually need is less.** You hold all of the wisdom, beauty, and power you need to find relief. And amid all of the noise, your connection to your body and nervous system are your most important teachers.

By taking a unique inside-out approach, this book is an empowering guide to help you understand that by going *inward*—into your body—and understanding your nervous system, you can make small but vital shifts that make living in a fast-paced, productivity-obsessed, and unsupportive culture more sustainable. The book blends supportive guidance with evidence-based research and tangible practices to offer a new paradigm for honoring our needs from a nervous-system-informed perspective.

Chapter 1 provides a language for the everyday ways our bodies communicate to us, including an accessible explanation of polyvagal theory and how we can activate our parasympathetic nervous system for ease and relief. In chapter 2, we begin the journey of learning how to assess our energy through nourishing tracking tools and how to honor our internal barometer and nervous system cues instead of overriding them. We will spend some time here connecting to and identifying our unmet needs, which are often a source of energy depletion. Finally, we will explore a number of practices for protecting the various dimensions of our energy. In chapter 3, I speak directly to those who are never able to hit the pause button. Through guided self-inquiry, you will be invited to reflect on what feels unsustainable and why, and envision a new way of showing up each day.

Chapter 4 explores the concept of embodied boundaries and the various ways stress and trauma can impact the nervous system. I'll introduce yogic philosophy and frameworks to show how setting boundaries and *embodying* them actually protects, and even heals, the nervous system. You will understand in essence why boundary work *is* nervous system work. In chapter 5, we delve into a mind-body-spirit approach to unwind from burnout, with a particular focus on how the highly sensitive nervous system is impacted.

Chapter 6 examines the various dimensions of rest, affirmations, and trauma-informed shapes you can explore when you are exhausted, offering a soft place to land as you begin to honor the various types of rest your nervous system needs. Chapter 7 expands upon those restorative frameworks and provides a range of micro self-care practices and trauma-informed meditations you can lean on during periods of overwhelm. In closing, you will be invited to reflect on what may be blooming in all of this new and open space and be reminded with so much love and care that sometimes our most important lessons arise from the stillness. Before engaging in any of these practices, and to confirm the source of your burnout, I urge you to consult your physician to look at your hormone health and blood panels, as your internal world can impact your mental and physical health, capacity, and well-being.

Throughout the book I have provided supportive guidance through reflection questions and journaling prompts that you can explore in your own time and at your own pace. You can also find a number of audio recordings of the trauma-informed meditations featured throughout the book at us.macmillan.com/ProtectYourEnergy or at this QR code.

As you work your way through the content and prompts offered to you, feel free to engage with them in any order you see fit. At any time, you can skip to the practices in chapters 6 and 7, explore the worksheets in the back of the book, or spend some time with the journaling prompts. Please make this your own sacred journey—whatever that looks like for you.

I want this book, more than anything else, to feel like a restorative exhale. I want you to have a place where you can feel seen and validated in all that you are carrying, a place where you can start to feel some relief. Before you move forward, I invite you to read the following gentle reminders and slowly reflect on what might be blooming or surfacing for you. Honor the pace of your breath and the rhythm of your heart as you do so.

- Boundary work is nervous system work.
- It is immensely necessary to take a break from the mental load of always "being on."
- It takes time to unwind from overworking.
- Often safety can feel like exhaustion because our bodies finally have permission to rest.
- There is a tangible joy in noticing what being grounded and at ease feels like in our bodies.
- There is beauty in not needing to strive for the next thing and instead feeling truly content right where we are.
- A deep love is able to emanate from within without timelines or deadlines.
- Having margins and boundaries in our day and not constantly responding to the urgency of others is powerful.
- Not rushing is so deeply healing and perhaps a love language all on its own.
- It's okay to *not* be in charge or take the lead on that thing. Really, I promise.
- It's important to not deflect the help and support we need and are worthy of when we are overwhelmed.
- It is so important to offer ourselves the compassion we so freely give to others.

- Our softness and sensitivity are our most powerful forms of strength.
- We are worthy of no longer putting our health as an afterthought.
- We have permission to release the pressure of getting everything done on today's list.
- The everyday intentional choices to protect our peace and honor our capacity have the potential to change our lives in radical ways.
- It is a very human response to need more rest during stressful seasons.
- We are worthy of reclaiming the parts of ourselves that have gotten lost in service to others.
- Having clarity around who has access to our energy is a profound practice.
- Our energy has a palpable impact on all those we love.
- In a world that will constantly demand more from us, being intentional and discerning with our energy is our most powerful resource.

We will revisit these anchors and gently unpack them more fully throughout the book because I am a firm believer that repetition, ritual, routine, predictability, and consistency can soothe and support those who might be struggling from a dysregulated nervous system. The evidence lies in the rituals of comfort you lean on in your own life, like your favorite playlist on repeat, that yoga sequence you always seem to go back to, the comfort show or movie you watch during hard times, your favorite comfortable cozy sweater, your favorite book that you pick back up every year, that yummy breakfast that always hits the spot, or the soul-nourishing rituals you start and end your day with.

They might seem simple and mundane, but these sacred rhythms are actually strengthening your neural pathways (neurons that send signals from one part of the brain to another) and offering you safety, control, and predictability when you need it most. According to Northwestern Medicine, predictable routines and rituals help ease anxiety, improve sleep, bring a sense of calm to the brain and body, reduce stress, and support emotional well-being and better mental health outcomes.[6] May we never underestimate the simplicity of these gifts to support the resilience and regulation of our nervous systems. When everything becomes too much, come back to the comforts that you know.

I hope that each time you come back to the various energy frameworks and practices repeatedly woven throughout the book, they land on your heart a little differently and perhaps remind you of what you need in the ebbs and flows of the particular season you are navigating. I hope they help you begin to nurture all the ways you are deserving of protecting your most precious resource: your energy.

Shifting our focus to managing our energy instead of our time has the potential to completely change our lives. When energy protection, bandwidth conservation, and mental health become the center, we can be more mindful about the everyday choices we make that help us show up for our lives with more fullness instead of constantly operating from states of depletion. This journey is also, of course, layered by our various life experiences. Trauma symptoms, chronic stress, and post-traumatic stress disorder (PTSD) are the body's way of communicating that we have undigested sensory residue that wants to be processed in some way (more on this in chapter 1). So as you learn more about what you might be navigating in your internal world, offer yourself the gift of self-compassion. While we can't fast-track our healing, we can celebrate the beauty of each brave new beginning.

You don't have to continue carrying it all and living in ways that deplete your energy. You can be mindful of the daily messages your body communicates to you and respond with kindness, compassion, and care. I hope the pages that follow inspire you through gentle, empowering, and evidence-based guidance. May you know that you are worthy of moving through your days with fullness instead of depletion, in ways that allow you to honor your capacity and protect your energy, and in ways that are expansive, fulfilling, and joyful. Together, we will work toward honoring your unique being and identifying a sustainable set of tools to support you. So cozy up with your softest clothes and blanket and maybe a warm beverage as you begin your journey back home to yourself.

Before moving on to chapter 1, I invite you to take a moment to explore the Nervous System Care Checklist in the additional resources section of this book. This worksheet was crafted to help set the foundation for the work we will do together and provides you with a number of tangible tools to tend to your nervous system. If you'd like, you can also access a PDF download at us.macmillan.com /ProtectYourEnergy or use this QR code.

1

Your Nervous System Is Your Friend and Teacher

To heal your nervous system, you must give yourself unconditional permission to relax. The damage caused by chronic stress can't be repaired by maintaining the same relentless pace that created it.[1]
—ABBY RAWLINSON

In my quietest moments, cozying up in my favorite chair on my front patio (with hot coffee in the mug I reach for everyday) and feeling a sliver of sun on my face to help thaw my bone-deep exhaustion, I often wonder how any of us manage the unsustainable pace of our lives. As I stare up at the clouds and listen to the birds, I find myself constantly dreaming of more creative and sustainable ways of being.

The way we move through our days depleted and in a constant state of urgency and exhaustion is not normal, but the greater systems that enfold us have made us believe it is. Most of us have come to accept this as reality, but it does not have to be. We are worthy of reclaiming our time and all of those lost choices. We are worthy of saying, "No, not like this." We are worthy of pausing and honoring our humanness and mental health instead of being expected to show up, pull it together, and power through. Why can't we celebrate pausing, resting, saying no, doing less, slowing down, and setting boundaries in the same way we celebrate hustle culture, constant achievement, overextending ourselves, and endless productivity? The relentless nature of being human is hard to escape, and none of us are immune from the next storm or our endless list of responsibilities. But I'm here to remind you that even amid it all, you are worthy of protecting your energy.

In her book *Polyvagal Exercises for Safety and Connection*, Deb Dana—clinician, consultant, author, and expert on polyvagal theory—shares that "among many experiences of dysregulation, there are also regularly occurring micro-moments of regulation, or glimmers" (which we will expand upon in this chapter). These tiny instances of calm include noticing the colors of the sunset, cuddling with a pet, reading a sweet text from a friend, taking advantage of unexpected space on your calendar, reveling in the company of someone's presence who feels like sunshine, and hearing a child's laugh. These simple moments allow us to redirect our energy and can have a profound impact on how we move through our days, experience more flow, and give our spirits the boost they need to get through.[2] And I don't mean this in a "spiritual bypassing" kind of way but rather in a way that honors all parts of ourselves and gives us the space and clarity to release the intense, frenetic pace and grip on "doing it all."

Many of us have been sold subtle messages about exhaustion and overscheduling from a young age. From early on, we may have been told that we need to bring our work home and have limited time for regulation, play, and decompression, lest this becomes a distraction from our academic success. It is no wonder so many adults struggle with work-life balance, perfectionism, and anxiety. As you begin the journey of intentionally protecting your energy, please know that you are chipping away at years of messaging and beginning to deprogram from the idea that your productivity is tied to your worth. With gentleness, awareness, patience, and time, you will come to realize that restoration, regulation, joy, and attunement to your body are accessible to you, even in small, bite-size ways.

Understanding this is one of the first steps toward befriending your nervous system and allowing it to be a teacher and guide to honoring your needs. When you take a scan of your life, what would doing less look like for you? What would it feel like? How might your life change? Let yourself linger in the answers and possibilities for as long as you'd like.

Cultivating a Nurturing Relationship with Your Nervous System

I've found that, so often, what prevents us from identifying ways life could feel even a *little* more manageable is the feeling of overwhelm. Without space for stillness, decompression, and integration, it can feel hard to access the answers we might be yearning for. One of the most affirming statements that I carry with me is one I saw on Instagram from body-positive speaker, feminist, and bestselling author Megan Jayne Crabbe that said, "You don't have to do the whole thing for it to count." This can apply to so many facets of life. Showing up for ourselves and getting started is often the hardest part. Honoring the fact that growth can feel painstakingly slow at times is challenging. Patience is healing. Once you begin the journey, the possibilities for reconceptualizing the space you take up in your life are endless. May we never underestimate the cumulative impact of the seemingly small ways we can begin to chip away at all that ails us.

Navigating multiple experiences of trauma and working in a trauma-informed field for over sixteen years has taught me a lot about my relationship to my own nervous system. I learned in many ways that my perfectionist tendencies to overwork, prepare tediously and relentlessly for countless work projects, and view everything through the lens of urgency were trauma responses that deserved healing. My relationship with my nervous system has ebbed and flowed and evolved in myriad and nonlinear ways, just as my healing journey has. The practice of tuning in to my nervous system, and listening to and honoring its messages, has helped buffer the more intense moments of my life. This was not a cure for grief or trauma, but it helped soften the edges and allow me to approach challenges and overwhelm from a place of fullness rather than depletion.

Cultivating a resilient nervous system allows us to process our stress, recalibrate, and flow more easily with life's daily stressors, so we don't get stuck in a sympathetic (fight-or-flight) state. This allows us to function and show up in our daily lives, be present, and move flexibly between our various nervous system states. As I began to chip away at the cumulative toll of stress and trauma that was living in my bones for years, the most compassionate practice I could offer myself was gentleness and grace.

Thanks to neuroplasticity (the rewiring of neural pathways), the practice became ingrained in my system over time and offered me space to navigate the storms that at times felt endless. I began to instinctively honor and tend to the most vulnerable parts of myself with an abundance of love and compassion. This in turn started to inform the way I spoke to myself when challenges or crises would arise. I eventually internalized that I was worthy of feeling the presence of peace in my life. Even saying that out loud brings all the emotions to the surface.

Take a moment here to reflect on your relationship with peace: how it shows up, what it feels like, how you cultivate it, and how you protect it. When I think about what peace feels like in my life, some of the first words that come to mind are spaciousness, ease, strong boundaries, and intentionality. A big part of cultivating more peace has been viewing asking for help as a form of strength and remembering the temporary nature of what I might be navigating in a particularly challenging season of life. Sometimes it helps me to do a guided meditation and visualize what my facial expressions look like when I feel at peace, what my environment looks like, and what I notice somatically in my nervous system (softness and lightness). I find it helpful to envision a warm light surrounding me and absorbing any barriers to my pathway to peace. My visions of peace don't have to be perfect, but giving myself the space to daydream about it makes it feel so much more tangible and attainable.

Lately I have been thinking about nervous system capacity, its intersection with preventative self-care (the ways we tend to ourselves *before* a busy time), and the amount of space I create for myself each day. Years of survival mode have programmed me to always wait for the next shoe to drop. The next crisis to arise. The next life event that would completely deflate me. Having my armor up all of the time in this way was exhausting, but it was part of how I kept myself "safe." It took time for me to cultivate another way of being.

A big part of nurturing flexibility in my nervous system is intentionally doing *less*, saying no, and taking things off of my plate.

Sometimes the hardest practice is actually learning how to do less and gently breaking patterns of overworking or numbing myself to avoid facing hard things. It takes courage to allow ourselves to feel deeply. It has taken self-compassion and intention to make this a daily preventative care practice in my life so I can avoid the aftermath of putting out fires in busy and trying seasons. Can you relate to this? Does doing less feel unrealistic to you?

The result of doing this energy-protection work is that it has allowed me to build resilience, so when those inevitable storms of life come along, I have more space to tend to them with groundedness and fluidity. The beauty of honoring the spectrum of our nervous system is that it helps prepare us to navigate the constant ebbs and flows of life. When we can remind ourselves often that nervous system regulation is about nurturing flexibility and resilience between our various physiological states instead of putting pressure on ourselves to be calm all the time, it can create noticeable shifts in our healing journey. How powerful of us to honor—without shame or stigma—all the ways our precious body communicates with us.

Just so we are clear, I *do not* have all the answers, and I still struggle to find my footing sometimes. One of the most self-affirming things we can do daily is to begin again with compassion and softness, which in my opinion is one of the most powerful forms of strength. How human of all of us to acknowledge just how challenging it is to pour into ourselves. And how brave of us to begin to carve out space to reclaim the in-between moments of our lives.

By cultivating an intentional relationship with your nervous system, you can reclaim control of the thousands of ways your energy is depleted each day. You may already be listening and attuning to the messages your body communicates to you in everyday moments: when you have an uncomfortable conversation and notice your face feels hot; when you feel joy and spaciousness and your whole system relaxes; when you spend time with someone you love and their presence makes you feel safe and at ease; when a stressful situation arises at work and you suddenly feel an overwhelming sense of urgency and a desire for control. ·

Continuing to cultivate this somatic attunement is how you begin to be in relationship with your energy and feel compelled to protect it. When you understand what activates your parasympathetic nervous system (the part of the nervous system that slows the heart and relaxes your muscles)[3] and center this as an everyday practice, you can more intentionally navigate each day in a way that's more easeful, restful, and sustainable. It is truly a beautiful and life-giving practice. The mind and body practitioners Jennifer Mann and Karden Rabin share "the goal in nervous system regulation is to rewire survival responses and maladaptive coping mechanisms and heal unresolved trauma pathways that have become our default states over time."[4] This rewiring helps decrease the toll that stress takes on the body.

So, here's to honoring our humanity and our changing capacity in the many seasons of life to come. This journey is about continuing to show up for yourself and remembering that you are worthy of giving your best versus your all. You deserve to have overflow and reserves for yourself and your loved ones. As the brain coach Jim Kwik reminds us, "On the days you only have 40 percent and you give 40 percent, you gave 100 percent."[5]

You are worthy of honoring your changing capacity.

You are worthy of honoring your changing capacity.

You are worthy of honoring your changing capacity.

You are worthy of honoring your changing capacity.

In this chapter, we will explore the relationship between energy and your nervous system by delving into what your exhaustion is communicating to you, the window of tolerance, polyvagal theory, our glimmers, the connection between energy and empathy, and most importantly how you can befriend your nervous system. I am so honored to explore this with you.

The Beginning

As a daughter of the most incredible, supportive, and hardworking immigrant parents, I grew up without having models of rest. Achieving was the norm, constantly packed schedules were how we functioned, and proving our worth to the outside world via our productivity was paramount. This is a common experience among children of immigrants. Many of us grow up with the pressure or desire to strive for "enoughness," only to realize that external validation will never be enough. The work needs to begin on the *inside*. It has taken me decades to unpack this narrative.

I recognize, with an outpour of self-compassion, all the ways this story impacted my habits, my patterns around overworking, my coping strategies, and my relationship with my nervous system. Combine this with years of working in toxic environments, being a survivor of multiple forms of trauma, identifying as a perfectionist and people pleaser, and having poor boundaries, and it's safe to say that the way I was living depleted me before I even had the language to describe or understand what was happening in my inner world.

It has taken time for me, as a survivor of trauma, to understand the difference between safety and danger. Living in constant states of hyperarousal for long periods of my life led to significant levels of energy depletion. The consistent and heightened sense of alertness made everything feel like a threat, which made resting feel unattainable. When people told me I just needed to practice "more self-care" or "find ways to rest," it actually felt triggering because I desperately wanted to, but my body cues, which were trying to protect me, were communicating otherwise. Those cues were hard to untangle from. But the cumulative toll of constantly overriding the cues of my nervous system eventually started to reveal itself. Listening to my body meant finding a unique and gentle path that honored the nuances of my lived experience.

In the height of the pandemic, while working full-time with no childcare, I ended up in the emergency room after a series of rolling panic attacks (one of the most vulnerable moments of my life). In that moment, my partner and I both knew that something needed to drastically change. Few words were exchanged; it was just a shared energy between us that signaled that another way had to be possible. And so began the slow and intentional journey of moving beyond survival and living my life outside of the crushing expectations of others—in ways that were community-oriented, boundless, expansive, and spacious. This was a place I had been yearning for but didn't know actually existed. It was tenderness embodied. It was a restorative exhale. It was a way to come back home to myself.

Prioritizing Your Energy

Prioritizing protecting my energy started to accumulate in larger ways. The more I listened to my body's signals, the more I trusted myself. The more I trusted myself, the more I believed in my innate worthiness. The more worthy I felt, the more aligned I became with my values and what aspects of my life deserved my yes. Slowly this process helped me become a priority in my life. Each of these things built upon the next. The beautiful part of growth is its subtleness, yet you can feel how palpable the impact is on your life. You are worthy of this feeling.

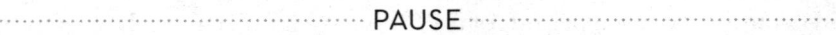

PAUSE

Journaling Prompts for Self-Reflection

I want to take a moment to acknowledge that so often our upbringing, environment, and life circumstances can deeply impact our habits and beliefs around centering our needs and caring for ourselves. This can be an emotional journey that requires our full participation and acknowledgment of the various experiences that have led us to this point.

For these reasons, I encourage you to spend some time with the following journaling prompts to take inventory of how you currently care for yourself and your nervous system. Honor what feels authentic for you and leave the rest. Hold yourself with care, pause when you need to, let the tears come, and know there is no need to judge yourself in this space. All parts of you, including your feelings and lived experiences, are welcome.

ON CAPACITY

- When you feel overwhelmed or are carrying a significant mental load, do you ask for and receive help from others? Is it hard for you to ask for help? What or who typically supports you during those particularly challenging moments of life?
- Is it hard for you to say no to taking on additional commitments, even when you don't have the bandwidth? If yes, how long has this been a pattern for you? What do you think is the root of this tendency?
- What is the quality of your energy like as you move and flow throughout your day? How often do you attune to your capacity? Did anyone ever model how to pay attention to and honor your energy levels? Is this a new concept for you?
- How often do you find yourself being the person who is in charge, taking the lead, or making plans? Can you remember how early you took on this role?

ON CARE

- How much space in your life do you create for yourself to simply do things you enjoy and that bring you pleasure?
- What is your relationship like with your mental and physical health? How often do you prioritize tending to these parts of yourself?
- Are you content with where you are in life or do you feel pressure to constantly strive for the next thing? Where do you feel these messages come from?
- Does your community know when you are struggling? Are you able to ask for support in a tangible way?

ON REST

- Growing up, did you have models of rest (people in your life who celebrated and honored rest as a daily practice)? How has this impacted your relationship with rest?

- Do you find ways to rest or downregulate throughout your day, or only at the end?
- Do you feel like you have to earn your rest? Do feelings of guilt arise when you do allow yourself to rest? Why do you think that is?
- Does rest feel restorative, or does it feel like collapse or failure? Why do you think that is the case?

ON WORK

- Reflect on the various types of work you do both inside and outside of the home. When you take a scan of what a typical week looks like for you, how do you usually feel? Full? Depleted? Energized? Exhausted? I encourage you to start tracking your experience without judgment. Be gentle with yourself here.
- How much of your identity is tied to what you do?
- Do you feel like you are always on and do you feel compelled to always be accomplishing things? Where in your life can you soften?

Once you've taken the time to reflect on these questions in your journal, take a moment to rest a palm over your belly and a palm over your heart. Explore your breath at your pace. There is absolutely no rush here. Feel into what these questions have brought up for you. Everything you are feeling is deeply valid.

·········· PAUSE ··········

Tending to Yourself with Care

These next few practices offer an opportunity for you to slow your pace and begin caring for your nervous system through the practices of self-tending and self-compassion. Choose one or more practices that feel most supportive for you and commit to integrating them into your daily life on a regular basis. Feel welcome to make the practices your own by exploring any variations of the invitations to increase your comfort. May they offer your nervous system a much-needed reset amid any moments of overwhelm.

- Rub your palms together to create warmth and then rest them over your heart. You deserve to take in your own compassion.
- Gently cradle the side of your face with your palm for a compassionate self-hold. Allow yourself to melt a little deeper into your care with each exhale. Take your time and be gentle with your experience.
- Find a sliver of sun and let it thaw any grief, stress, or tension you may be holding in your body. Notice where you might feel even a small sense of softening. You are doing an amazing job.
- Rest a palm over your heart and a palm over your belly if that feels supportive for you. As best as you can, explore quieting your mind by envisioning that you are turning the volume of your heart all the way up and the volume of your thoughts all the way down. Notice the rise and fall of your beautiful, powerful breath. Follow the unique pace of your nervous system.
- On your inhale, draw your shoulders up; on your exhale, release them back and down your spine. For a moment and within the container of this space, release whatever you have been carrying. You are worthy.
- Take some time to connect to the parts of you that need a little extra support and care. You might massage your temples, the back of your head and shoulders, and/or your earlobes. Take your time; there is no rush.
- Interlace your fingers and extend your hands up toward the sky. Invite gentle side bends if that feels good for you.

Your Nervous System and You

Ease up some of that burden you put on
yourself, love. One foot in front of the other.
Small steps, every day, will add up.[6]
—WE THE URBAN

A TENDER NOTE

The invitation is to read this section slowly, as there is a lot
of information to unpack as it relates to your unique relationship with your nervous system. Please honor your lived
experience, go slow, take breaks, and release the pressure
to digest this information quickly.

On a daily basis, we are fluidly switching between the sympathetic
nervous system (SNS)—a network of nerves that engages when the
body is stressed, activated, in danger, or physically active—and the parasympathetic nervous system (PNS)—a network of nerves that helps
restore and relax the body to a sense of calm. This is a normal part
of being human, and it's natural to experience these ebbs and flows
throughout the day. For instance, you might sit down with a cup of
tea and a warm blanket to decompress (activating your PNS) and then
get jolted out of your reverie by the doorbell ringing and your dog
barking (activating your SNS). These ebbs and flows help us cultivate
resilience and flexibility within our nervous system.

However, as we have begun to explore together, when we exist
in consistent states of hyperarousal (increased physical sensations,
hypervigilance, or anxiety), it can become incredibly challenging
to switch off the sympathetic nervous system and settle ourselves.
This is the quickest road to energy depletion, nervous system dysregulation, and physical symptoms of stress, such as stomach pains,
migraines, and more.

This is why our goal is to find spaces of calm and safety through-out our days so we can intentionally activate our parasympathetic nervous system. This allows us to ease back into a relaxation response, which supports our recovery from stress.[7] Nervous system practices can support us with daily downregulation strategies as well as temper physiological symptoms.

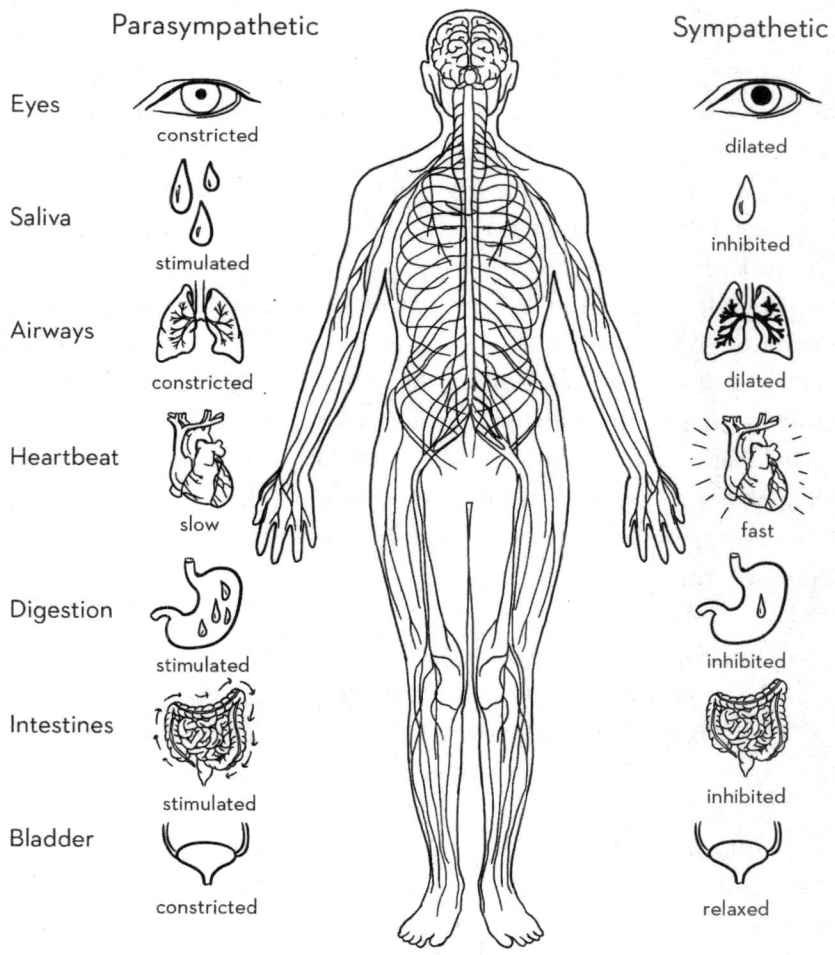

The parasympathetic and sympathetic nervous systems affect various organs throughout the body.

So often the various symptoms we experience or protective strategies we use to relieve ourselves from these stressful states are somatic reenactments of past trauma. For example, we may dissociate as a way to help us create a safe container because what we are currently managing in our lives is overwhelming to our nervous systems. Or maybe we feel overtaxed, and as our bodies work to do their best with the resources available, we experience headaches. Stress and overwhelm impact all parts of us—physical, emotional, mental, social, and spiritual—which is why we often have a hard time compartmentalizing the way we experience them. But you are worthy of honoring—without shame or stigma—all the ways your body has supported your survival. Let this become an embodied reminder that your worthiness is not up for negotiation, and you are inherently whole.

When we navigate life on high alert all of the time, it can be challenging for rest to actually *feel* restorative. Sometimes it may feel more like collapse. Even as we start the process of cultivating safety within ourselves, it is normal to still feel exhausted. The psychotherapist Meg Josephson shares, "If the body has been in a state of hypervigilance for days, months, years, or decades, that means the body has been running on high levels of cortisol and adrenaline, which it's not meant to do for that amount of time. It takes time for the body to recover and recuperate and get used to this new feeling of safety."[8] Healing takes time, love, so give yourself grace if your attempts at doing less don't feel so restful at first.

> *Sometimes safety can feel like exhaustion because your body finally has permission to rest. Be so very gentle with yourself. All of your chapters of healing are worthy of compassion and care.*

This brings us back to that earlier question about the presence of peace and calm in your life. If it feels unattainable right now, it is okay. You don't need additional pressure on yourself. You deserve compassion and affirmation right where you are. May you know, feel, and believe that it will not always be this hard. Practice patience with your experience as you take in new information. The insights you gain may provide context and affirmation to something you have been navigating for quite some time. You are seen and supported through it all.

If it all feels like a bit too much, the window of tolerance offers us a holistic way to take in all of this information in a digestible way and begin the process of integration in our lives.

The Window of Tolerance

The window of tolerance, a concept that was developed by Dr. Daniel J. Siegel, is often used in trauma theory to help us understand how our bodies respond to stress. It typically refers to the "sweet spot" in our emotional state, where we feel most at ease. This concept empowers us to attune to the physiological states in our bodies so we can build awareness around when we might be moving into various nervous system states—*without judgment*—and broaden our window of tolerance. You don't need to feel any shame for the way your body communicates with you. As best as you can, try to view all bodily sensations and emotions as information.

It can be comforting to name and understand when there might be a buildup of residue from stress or trauma accumulating in our bodies, depending on what we might be experiencing or navigating on any given day. There is power in this kind of nonjudgmental awareness because it can inform the steps we take or the support we lean on in order to feel some relief. It also allows us to reconceptualize our experiences through the lens of a continuum and understand that we have the ability to access tools to shift our nervous system states. The key is finding and applying the right practices for *your* unique nervous system.

As you look at this visual, I encourage you to take a baseline of your general nervous system states. How do you feel when you are experiencing hyperarousal, or heightened anxiety? Anxious? On edge? Irritable? Do you struggle to get into a flow state or feel connected to others? Do you experience panic or extreme worry? Alternatively, how do you feel when you are experiencing hypoarousal, or a state

The Window of Tolerance

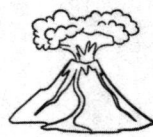

Hyperarousal

- You feel anxious, angry, or out of control.
- You may want to fight or run away.
- You are in an abnormal state of increased responsiveness.

Dysregulation

- You may start to feel agitated, anxious, or angry.
- You do not feel comfortable, but you are not out of control yet.

Shrink
your window
of tolerance

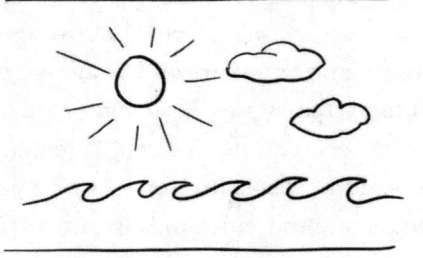

Expand
your window
of tolerance

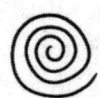

Dysregulation

- You may start to feel overwhelmed, and your body may start shutting down. You may begin to lose track of time.
- You do not feel comfortable, but you are not out of control yet.

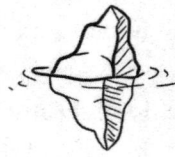

Hypoarousal

- You are in an abnormal state of decreased responsiveness.
- You feel emotional numbness, exhaustion, or depression.
- You may experience your body shutting down or freezing.

The window of tolerance

of underwhelm? Numb, depressed, disconnected? A lack of energy? Do you shut down or dissociate?

Additionally, we can certainly experience subtler examples of dysregulation on this continuum. For example, we may feel irritable and headed toward hyperarousal but stop short of experiencing a full-on panic attack. Alternatively, we may experience moments in our day where we are deeply exhausted and perhaps headed toward hypoarousal, but we may not experience full dissociation. Ideally, as we start to tune in more deeply to the sensations our bodies communicate to us in these moments of dysregulation, we can intervene with supportive practices. By doing so, the pendulum won't swing so far to our edges that it makes it harder to get back to our window of tolerance.

When you are in your window of tolerance or your unique and sacred "sweet spot," you might feel an increased ability to be present. You might have more capacity to handle daily stressors; feel safe, content, and joyful; and have space to be compassionate with yourself and others. You may also notice that you feel more connected, regulated, in flow, grounded, and spacious. This is also known as a ventral vagal state, which we will build upon in the next section.

I know it is tempting to want to shift your nervous system states right away, and you might feel pressure to find quick fixes on your healing journey. I can empathize deeply with wanting instant relief. But the most important thing I want to affirm is the power of first honoring where you are in this moment without taking on any added self-blame. When we can offer ourselves grace for all we have navigated that has led us to now, it can help us soften and humanize our experience. From this place we can start to do the hard but powerful internal work of healing our nervous system from the inside out. With the support of the practices and frameworks in this book, I am confident you will start to find the pockets of relief you have been yearning for and gain strategies for widening your window of tolerance and cultivating a healthy, resilient, and flexible nervous system.

For example, if you notice you are headed toward hyperarousal, you could give yourself space from your phone or emails to limit any more overstimulation, go for a walk or do some other movement to help complete your stress cycle (more on this in chapter 5), or ask for tangible support amid the overwhelm. If you notice you are headed toward hypoarousal, you might focus on small tasks such as brushing your teeth, making your bed, stretching, breathing, or sitting in the sun to thaw any grief or tension that might be present. The more you become familiar with what works for you, the more these practices will start to feel like the sacred rituals they are. You may even start to lean into preventative self-care practices where you take care of yourself *before* you reach states of dysregulation.

As you move through the practices in this book, I invite you to track with an abundance of care and gentleness which tools and frameworks of care feel most soothing to your nervous system and increase your margins of rest. There is no one-size-fits-all approach, so start to notice what you gravitate toward and what resonates most with your heart. This awareness will help you compassionately connect your mind, body, and spirit amid all of the disintegration that stress and trauma can cause, so you can widen your window of tolerance over time and settle your nervous system.

What follows are a few examples of how my typical morning activities getting the kids ready for school might affect my nervous system on any particular day, depending on the various stressors I am navigating in my life, how much sleep I have gotten, or the type of support I can access. My hope is that these examples demonstrate how we are subtly (or not so subtly) affected by our normal day-to-day activities, and so help you generate more awareness. Hold all of this with a compassionate lens and remember that your best will look different every day. We can't always anticipate the curveballs we may experience on any given week or the constant factors that impact our energy and capacity. I encourage you to take some time throughout your week to reflect in a similar way on how you're feeling and decide if your experiences fall into any of these categories.

Hyperarousal: Today I felt totally overwhelmed. I felt like I was spiraling, and I needed to escape into my room for a few moments while my heart was racing. I could feel the onset of a panic attack. I felt incredibly rushed and anxious when thinking about my work deadlines as I was trying to get the kids ready for school and out the door. I felt extremely irritable and stressed.

Dysregulation: I started to notice anxious and irritable feelings arising as I was rushing to gather the kids' belongings. To combat this, I tried slowing the pace of my breath.

Window of Tolerance: Today I felt grounded, at ease, and able to move swiftly through the various tasks of the morning. I felt joy being present with the kids and getting them to school, and I paused to connect with and hug my husband instead of rushing past him. I was honest with my staff about my capacity and boundaries, and I felt spaciousness in my day. I asked a family member for help since I knew it was going to be a full week, and I prioritized time for myself by getting coffee with a friend and going to my favorite yoga class. In general I felt content, a warm feeling in my heart, and better equipped to handle the stressors of the day.

Dysregulation: I felt unmotivated this morning, and it was harder to get up and move through my tasks. I splashed some water on my face and allowed myself to move slower than I usually do.

Hypoarousal: Today I felt completely frozen, dissociated, and unable to function. Even seemingly minor tasks felt incredibly overwhelming. I experienced brain fog and felt deeply exhausted. After the kids went to school, I couldn't get out of bed.

If you find that your daily routines often leave you in a state of dysregulation, I want to affirm for you that hope is on the other side. Cultivating a relationship with your body and understanding the various ways it has been impacted by trauma or chronic stress can be one of the most validating experiences because it helps you begin to understand your unique and nuanced relationship to your most precious resource: *yourself*. As you move through this process and build attunement to your needs, you will start to get a sense of what activates your parasympathetic (relaxed) nervous system throughout your day and slowly notice where you feel more flow and rest.

For example, you may learn the power and impact of intentional choices, such as closing your eyes for a few moments instead of reaching for your phone to scroll or sitting down on the couch to daydream instead of putting pressure on yourself to complete more tasks. Over time and with repetition, these new patterns will soften your overstimulation, give you space that may have otherwise felt unattainable, and support you with building new neural pathways that ground you in your worth. The subtle, gentle, and nourishing shifts to reclaim your energy await you.

> **GENTLE REMINDER**
>
> Sometimes a sea of other people's voices can move us further from our own. When you are in search of ways to calm and center yourself, may you remember and connect to your innermost voice, which is truly the most sacred. You are the integration. You are the teacher. You are the magic.

······································ PAUSE ·······································

An Embodied Practice for Containment

Sometimes we experience emotions or events that are too much for us to handle in the moment. While it's always best to let these heavy feelings pass through our bodies, we may have to put them aside for a little while until we are in a better space to engage with them intentionally. In this exercise, you will explore a practice of containment, which allows you to temporarily store distressing or overwhelming feelings and return to them later when you have more capacity and space to process or unpack them.

If you are able, I invite you to come into a Warrior I (Virabhadrasana I) shape. Starting in a standing posture, bring your right foot to the front of your mat, slightly bending your right knee if that feels comfortable. Bring your left foot to the back of your mat, placing it parallel to the back edge of the mat. Point your left hip forward and your right hip back, and rest for a moment in this posture. Feel free to make any adjustments or variations to increase your comfort.

From here, inhale and extend your arms high to the sky, drawing energy and intention through your fingertips. On your exhale, push your palms out and away from your body. This is a symbolic gesture of protecting your energy and creating space for what feels heavy. If this shape is inaccessible, feel free to explore the hand motions from a seated position.

Take note of the difference between absorbing and observing whatever might feel heavy for you. Even if just for a moment, you can temporarily release it and envision more space opening up within you until you have more capacity to be with it. You might envision you are placing the feeling or experience in a solid box or something else that makes room for what you're feeling. Be gentle with yourself here.

Continue this expression of moving the energy out and away from your body. You can always come back to this exercise when your nervous system feels regulated and flexible enough to tend to anything that might feel activating or overwhelming. For now, you are giving yourself the space you need.

The Vagus Nerve

The vagus nerve and polyvagal theory offer an accessible way for you to relate and tend to your inner world with care and compassion. The vagus nerve is our tenth cranial nerve in a "family of neural pathways" that wander throughout the body.[9] It operates independently of the spinal cord and wanders from the brain stem to the organs of the body to calm them down. It is essentially our rest-and-digest nerve. Most importantly, it helps us understand the interconnection between our gut and our emotional state, playing an instrumental role in the expression of emotions in our body. When we learn to stimulate it, the vagus nerve can help us manage a variety of psychosomatic symptoms.

When we feel unsafe, our sympathetic state may be activated, which may create consistent feelings of dysregulation that manifest as different symptoms, like eye twitching, overstimulation, anxious thoughts, and deep exhaustion (just to name a few). In this state, experiences might feel quite intense, and navigating your days can feel somewhat like a swinging pendulum. When we feel safe, on the other hand, the ventral branch of the vagus nerve supports our ability to feel calm and access rest—what's known as the ventral vagal state. This state is what allows us to find flow, space, and ease.

Yoga and similar movement or embodiment-based practices help stimulate the vagus nerve, address physiological imbalances, and rewire and repattern the nervous system, which supports our overall health and well-being.[10] Learning how to actively downregulate your nervous system into ventral vagal states throughout your day can help you access greater depths of inner capacity, groundedness, and resilience. When you are able to more consistently access this state, you reduce the chances of your nervous system being hijacked in the face of crisis or daily challenges and stressors, like irritating emails, uncomfortable phone calls, or road rage.

Although it sounds complex, activating a ventral vagal state doesn't have to be complicated. There are simple exercises and practices you can do as often as you'd like to help you soften, calm your nervous system, and prevent distressing feelings. The following practices are wonderful ways to protect and reclaim your energy. Take note of which of these speak to you and try to incorporate them throughout your day.

- Supportive social engagement and social connection
- Trauma-sensitive breathwork
- Walking
- Slowness and releasing urgency

- Time in nature
- Taking note and tracking experiences of awe and wonder
- Journaling
- Butterfly hug and soothing self-compassion holds (more on this in chapter 7)
- Meditation
- Stretching
- Restorative yoga
- Eating nourishing meals
- Sleeping
- Creating an emotional safety ritual
- Any type of movement that brings you joy
- Creativity
- Grounding practices

In her book *Reclaiming You*, the therapist Abby Rawlinson shares ten signs that signal you are in the ventral, safe-and-social state:

1. You feel safe, calm and present
2. You have a general sense of "everything is OK"
3. You can be productive and creative
4. You feel comfortable and secure being in your own company or being with others
5. You feel clear-headed and able to focus
6. You feel capable of handling whatever comes your way
7. You trust yourself and the world around you
8. You are able to collaborate with others
9. Your thoughts tend to be compassionate and curious, rather than critical and rigid
10. You can be organized and follow through with plans.[11]

These examples provide a comprehensive way for us to know when we are in our expanded window-of-tolerance state and how we can grow our capacity by protecting our energy. There was a time in my life when I had to tap into these practices daily to activate my ventral vagal state in order to keep myself grounded and centered.

I still remember the exact moment I got the call from my husband that after multiple tests and opinions, he had a cancerous tumor in his neck that had been undiagnosed for thirty years and had completely encased his facial nerve. This would require intensive surgery, radiation, and a number of postsurgical treatments to support his recovery and care. I was driving to yoga when I received the news and began crying hysterically. Although my heart was shattered into a million pieces, something within me knew that my nervous system needed that class. I arrived to my mat and let the tears fall while I laid in a fetal position for most of the practice. The teacher tended to my heart with the utmost respect and care and held space for my experience just as it was.

Trauma is familiar to me, but there was something different about the groundedness I felt as I held space for my husband throughout that time in our life. It did not "take me out" the way other crises have in the past, and I was able to draw from my reservoir and capacity because of the everyday work I put into my care. (I promise you it adds up when you need it most.)

With the help of yoga and my tool kit of embodiment practices, I was able to move through the process with my husband and make informed decisions around advocacy. Of course I wasn't immune from feeling overwhelmed or terrified or asking "Why us?" but my nervous system had a little more stability and flexibility to tend to the various layers of that life experience. I thank the universe daily that my husband is healthy and strong and for the resilience that carried us through more challenges than we ever imagined possible. I want the same for you as you nurture your connection to your nervous system, body, and overall energy.

·· PAUSE ··

A Moment of Embodied Connection and Practice

For a moment, and within the safety and container of this space, I invite you to gently connect to the wisdom of your nervous system by finding any shape of rest that feels supportive, accessible, and nourishing in your body. Take all the time you need and take up all the space you deserve.

Feel free to take a few moments to set up your space, whether indoors or outdoors, in a way that feels supportive and compassionate. Perhaps that means reaching for a pillow or bolster, an extra blanket, or an eye pillow—anything that would allow you to tend to your needs with care and intention. You are welcome to keep your eyes open, closed, or find a soft gaze. You are free to do what feels best for you. The choices you make with your body are absolutely celebrated in this space.

There is no need to strive or push in this space. *You are enough just as you are now.* In this moment, tend to your relationship with rest and take notice of what is asking to come to the surface. Everything you are feeling is valid and welcome here. Invite in a sacred pause and a deeper and braver breath. A moment to ground and be present with your experience. Let everything you have been carrying roll off of your shoulders and into the space that holds you here today.

Notice where you feel ease or constriction. Can you shift your body in a way that makes yourself even 5 percent more comfortable? You might decide to rest a palm over your heart and a palm over your belly and notice the rise and fall of your beautiful, powerful breath. Perhaps you'll explore turning the volume of your heart up and the volume of your thoughts all the way down. Or maybe you find comfort in gently circling your palm at your heart, engaging with this soothing motion for as long as it feels good for you.

As you settle deeper and deeper in this space, I invite you to gently orient yourself here. Take a moment to notice the support beneath you, whether it's a chair, a mat, or the soles of your feet. Take some time to embody what it feels like to be held amid all of the holding that you do each day. Know that you are strong and supported. You are never alone in your experience.

Take a scan around your space and notice what brings you a sense of ease. It might be gazing out the window at nature, cuddling with a pet, or taking a sip of water. If you can feel the sun, I invite you to release any tension in your shoulders and place your attention on the feeling of the sun on any parts of your body that need care and support. You might envision that the sun is helping to soften and thaw any areas where tension, trauma, or grief might be held. Let a visualization come to mind that feels supportive to your needs.

Can you trust the strength of your body to hold you here? Can you honor what freedom feels like in your body? Stay in this space of ease and rest for as long as it feels comfortable. There is no rush. When you are ready, gently invite movement back into your body. If you're willing and able, rub your palms together to create a sense of warmth and then rest them over your heart. Take some time to linger here in your own compassion and rest in this space of groundedness and calm.

To access an audio recording of this meditation,
visit us.macmillan.com/ProtectYourEnergy.

What Your Exhaustion Is Communicating to You

In a world that glamorizes "big breakthroughs,"
the truth is that most of the healing work
actually lies in the small, slow, tedious, digestible
process of showing up for ourselves over
and over and over again. Keep going.[12]
—THAÍS SKY

I have the words of this epigraph on a sticky note in my office, and I read them every day because repetition and consistency support embodiment. And embodiment is more attainable when we give ourselves space, grace, and time to process and integrate what we are feeling.

I imagine many of you might be reading this and thinking, *But how is it possible to center my needs with everything I am currently carrying?* Those of us who are navigating persistent demands, burnout, the impacts of systemic oppression and toxic capitalism, trauma, and the nonlinear journey of healing may feel like survival mode is the only option. But living this way can lead to something called adrenal fatigue—a chronic, body-wide state of exhaustion.

Our adrenals regulate the level of cortisol (stress hormone) in our bodies, and when this system is working in excess, constantly pumping out cortisol in response to stressful environments, adrenal fatigue can occur, ultimately leading to a multitude of health impacts, including anxiety, depression, and chronic fatigue, where even seemingly small tasks feel incredibly overwhelming.

If this sounds like your current reality, I see you. Luckily there are ways you can find some relief and give your nervous system a break. Let's try a quick exercise now. I encourage you to invite movement into your body in whatever way feels natural, supportive, and accessible at this moment. Perhaps you can do some neck rolls, finding a half circle or full circle and switching sides whenever you feel ready. Or you can gently rub your palms together to create a little warmth and offer a self-massage to any parts of you that need care and attention, like the back of your shoulders, your temples, your earlobes, your eyelids, or your forearms. Take all the time you need here; there is no rush. Your nervous system is worthy of your care.

While we can't shed all of our daily responsibilities, and while we cannot (at least not right now) completely eliminate the systems that consistently oppress us, what we can do is *tend* to ourselves and our internal landscape with the compassion it deserves. But it takes radical courage and vulnerability to do so. This is the path to our own care, worth, and liberation—one we can return to over and over again as much as we need. This path that will ultimately lead you to a softer connection with yourself.

I wish I could tell you there were quick fixes for immediate relief, but true, lasting healing requires a slow, internal shift in the way you prioritize yourself in your life and protect your precious energy. It'll show in the way you start to view setting boundaries as a sacred practice and in the way you begin to gently release the unrealistic expectations that others place on you. Over time, these consistent practices will create shifts that feel like a gentle, embodied joy. Like the feeling you get when the sun peeks through the trees or when the ocean breeze kisses your face. You will notice the moments that make you feel more alive and awake to your life.

As you move through the rest of the book and begin unpacking the various layers of what might be depleting your energy, I invite you to offer yourself the compassion you would give to a beloved person in your life. This is a brave journey. As the author and poet Brianna Pastor so beautifully puts it, "You can still make a beautiful life for yourself even if you lost many years of it to grief, darkness, or a wound that wouldn't close."[13]

The very nature of our current society makes it incredibly challenging to have spaciousness and buffers of care in our days. The constant striving and tasking programmed into us only adds to the personal burdens and pressures that so many humans carry. We deserve so much more than simply trying to get by and survive. We deserve more than this perpetual feeling of exhaustion.

Think about how many times you have replied "I am so tired" when someone asks how you are doing. Surely this could point to actual exhaustion, but it's likely it could also mean:

- I don't have the support I need.
- My workload is too much.
- I find it challenging to rest.
- I have unmet needs.
- I don't feel seen or validated for the mental load I am carrying.
- I am experiencing depression and anxiety.
- My mind, body, and spirit are taxed from constant demands.
- I don't have time to practice self-care.
- I am unable to take a break from caretaking.

Whether you realize you're doing it or not, existing in overdrive and survival mode drains all types of energy: physical, mental, emotional, and even spiritual (more on this in chapter 2). As Tricia Hersey, the founder of the Nap Ministry, reminds us constantly, "Rest is a radical act of resistance."[14]

When you're feeling this bone-deep exhaustion, I invite you to affirm to yourself: *I intentionally work toward releasing the grip that survival mode has on my heart. I invite in more ease, compassion, grace, and restoration to my spirit. I am not alone in this journey. My best is always enough.*

Take Your Joy Seriously and Find the Glimmers

Don't postpone or reschedule your joy.

The writer Kimani Fambro once said, "My joy is never a coincidence; I do the work."[15] We don't always hear it framed this way, but *joy is a practice*. In her book *Choose Joy*, the positive psychology practitioner Sophie Cliff explains the correlation between cultivating joy and burnout prevention. She shares how when we immerse ourselves in whatever brings us joy, "we give our brains and bodies a break from the cortisol released when we feel stressed or under pressure."[16] She also identifies some core, research-based foundations of joy, which include connection, experiences over things, savoring, movement, practicing kindness, lifelong learning, and creativity.[17] In other words, it's important to be intentional with your joy because it might be the very thing that allows your body to finally relax.

Savoring joy has become an integral practice in my life. Hardship, trauma, and stress can sometimes make it hard to be present with what is actually going well, especially if crisis always feels inevitable. But I want to remind you that you have the power to take note of the simple but extraordinary moments of your life. **Celebration shouldn't only be saved for big milestones. Everyday healing and living is something to celebrate too.**

I encourage you to envision your joy as a ball of light that you hold with the utmost care and intention in the palms of your hands. Romanticize it. Hold it tenderly. And celebrate even the tiniest joys that bring your nervous system ease, care, and safety. This practice can become a lifeline during life's storms.

In addition to Cliff's influence, I started to become intentional about savoring subtle and energetic moments of joy after I began a practice that Deb Dana describes as "finding the glimmers." Glimmers are "micro-moments of ventral experience that routinely appear in everyday life yet frequently go unnoticed. A glimmer could be seeing a friendly face, hearing a soothing sound, or noticing something in the environment that makes you smile."[18] Glimmers are a powerful tool for filling your cup and adding to your energy in a world that constantly tries to drain it. Over time, these micro-moments accumulate and help provide a reservoir for your energy that you can tap into at any time.

Helen Marie, a therapist and author of *Choose You*, offers the most beautiful breakdown of glimmers. "Glimmers are the opposite of triggers," she says:

- they are tiny moments of awe
- they spark joy & evoke inner calm
- they have a positive effect on our mental health
- they are micro-moments causing tiny mood shifts
- they send cues of safety to our nervous system
- they bring feelings of ease & contentment
- our body responds with positive energy
- they allow us to feel hope when lost
- our nervous system is strengthened by them
- they can help increase our well-being
- once we start embracing them, it can become a beautiful way to see the world around you.[19]

Glimmers provide a way for us to intentionally activate our parasympathetic nervous system because when we fully drop into a moment of ease or joy with the full senses of our mind, body, and spirit, our whole system is able to relax. I know I often take these simple moments of regulation for granted because the stress can feel loud, fiery, and overpowering. But other times, just the awareness of them has the ability to make a subtle yet profound shift in my mood.

For example, while working on my manuscript and feeling looming deadlines, my son asked if I could cuddle with him. The sweetness of that sacred moment of co-regulation boosted my serotonin levels and helped create so much spaciousness that I was able to come back to my work with a renewed spirit. There was another moment when my son noticed the distressed look on my face, then closed my laptop and said, "It's okay, Mama. It doesn't have to be perfect." What a profound reminder for us all.

In your journal, take a moment to reflect on the glimmers that may be in your immediate space or recall any you may have experienced today but perhaps weren't able to pay much attention to in the moment. I invite you to take in the fullness of these moments and notice what sensations arise in your body because of them. Take your time. The goal is to practice not just the awareness but the *embodiment*. As you move through your days, I encourage you to start cultivating your own glimmers practice and take note of how these moments feel in your body and how they directly impact your energy. Perhaps your glimmers give you a palpable sense of relief in your shoulders, a feeling of embodied joy, a noticeable decrease in your stress levels, an increased sense of connection and warmth, or a growing capacity in your heart for feelings of contentment.

By understanding your nervous system, you can begin to attune to your physiology and let it guide you to live your life in a way that is more grounded, purposeful, sustainable, and joyful. In the next chapter, we will start to get more practical about how to assess and protect your energy. I know when I am struggling with honoring myself and my needs, beginning with tangible practices and reminders can often ground me in the journey ahead and give me some semblance of control. Let's start to unpack what it means to protect your energy.

2

How to Assess and Protect Your Energy

I wasted a lot of energy over the years staying
in spaces where I thought, if I could just show
to this person or these people my light and my
heart and value, they would reciprocate the
energy. Lesson: Your worth is not predicated on
whether or not others can recognize it in you.[1]
—JOÉL LEON

Have you ever walked into a space where your intuition communicated that the vibes were off? It might have been hard to put it into words, but you could feel a palpable shift. That was your innate energy detector. Energy is something we give and receive. It is something that can be cultivated or drained, and it is communicated in so many ways: through our body language, our shortness or irritability, our supportive presence, our softening and ability to be a source of co-regulation for another human, our safe touch, and much more. Although it's hard to describe in words, when we take care of our energy, it has a ripple effect as we move through the world. Perhaps that's what adds to its preciousness. And because energy is so integral to the way we show up each day and a powerful way to shape the spaces we are in, we must be mindful of how we steward it.

Increase Your Margins

Unfortunately, our energy can also be easily depleted because so often our nature is to be reckless with it. My gentle invitation to you is to stop being reckless with your energy. I realize this is much easier said than done. In a single day, we may be navigating sleep deprivation; caregiving for young children, aging elders, or both; coping with stress from interactions with a toxic boss or employer; relentlessly tragic news cycles and the corresponding feeling of heartbreak and helplessness; and a seemingly never-ending to-do list. All of this can offer a clear visual of how little energy reserves may be available to us in any given moment, which can show up in our body as the inverse of glimmers, such as constriction and the inability to notice joy. As my beautiful friend and colleague Azita Nahai always reminds me, "There is so much joy that is trapped inside." We may even be doing "all" of the things to care for our mental health and tend to ourselves, and yet we still might be struggling. You are not alone. As we've learned so far, what the nervous system often needs is *less*.

The intense moments, interactions, and experiences that we navigate each day can take up a lot of real estate in our minds, bodies, and spirits, turning into a recurrent cycle of depletion that impedes our ability to focus on the things that actually replenish our energy. Calling our attention back to ourselves as a daily practice and priority is how we reclaim our energy and power.

Whenever someone shares with me that they are feeling overwhelmed or depleted, I of course always validate and affirm their experience and create space for them to be with all of their feelings just as they are. One of the first concepts I invite them to explore is "increasing their margins," which means building transitions and more space into their days. When we increase the margins in our day, we give ourselves buffers between tasks, create time to decompress, integrate rest as a daily practice, ask for and receive support, honor the space we need from relationships that exhaust us, and give ourselves room to process whatever might be showing up. This approach can help us nurture our schedule as best as we can with intention and in ways that honor our capacity instead of trying to operate at a machinelike pace devoid of human feeling.

I wonder how much might shift in our lives if we all softened our desire for perfection and turned down the pressure of the expectations we place on ourselves. The more information we have about our habits, coping strategies, and daily stressors, the more we can start to intentionally center our needs and protect our energy. I invite you to think about the ways you might increase your margins and lower expectations for your labor. For example, maybe you'll choose not to run that extra errand or not answer that phone call after a long day. You are worthy of delegating, asking for support, not taking the lead, saying no, not having all of the answers, not responding right away, and not getting sucked into the urgency of others.

In addition to making space in our lives for moments of reprieve, by increasing our margins, we also get to constantly redefine what success looks like for us. From a young age, I always thought success meant "climbing the ladder," achieving all of the things, and being in a constant state of striving. Of course, there is nothing wrong with wanting these things, but as I have begun trusting the ebbs and flows of my healing journey and my energy, I've started to be intentional about reconceptualizing what success actually means for me versus what I've been told it should mean. I am also more attuned to the fact that our definitions of success can shift in different stages and seasons of life.

These days, success for me looks like having time in the morning to be present with my kids, prioritizing my well-being instead of having it be an afterthought, building more flexibility in my schedule, setting boundaries around how much energy and space work takes up (a huge shift for a recovering workaholic), scheduling dates with friends and time for fun, and saying no to projects that might be exciting but would be depleting. If this sounds familiar to you, it's because it is! My idea of success now is closely intertwined with my needs instead of what I had been taught to want.

We all deserve to be in an evolving relationship with success. Amber Lyon, the author of *You Are a Magnet*, encourages us to reconsider the importance we place on "external success vs. the internal success available to us in this moment."[2] It can be as simple as wanting more peace in our lives and grinding less, striving for more presence with loved ones and rushing less, or building in more boundaries and giving in to fewer distractions. We can give ourselves permission to find a pace of life that best meets our needs and helps us tend to our internal world with intention and kindness. We can gently release the constant striving in small, accessible ways if it's not serving us. I encourage you to reflect on what success currently looks like for you and how that differs from what you've been taught to want or strive for. The answers might surprise you!

GENTLE REMINDER

You deserve to protect your time, schedule, energy, and spirit. You are worthy of presence, pleasure, wholeness, fun, and joy. You are more than your exhaustion.

Energy, Empathy, and Compassion for Others

> Making someone feel seen, heard, and
> understood is the loudest way to love them.[3]
> —WILDFAITH

I started this chapter by inviting you to reflect on a time when the vibes in the room felt off. Alternatively, have you ever walked away from an interaction with someone and thought to yourself, *That person has really good energy?* That could mean so many different things to you, but it often communicates that you felt seen, safe, cared for, nourished, and generally good in their presence. Perhaps they exuded or embodied a warmth that added levity to your day. Maybe the interaction gave you an energy boost that created a ripple effect as you moved into interactions with others. Can you recall a moment where you've experienced this? As they say, energy doesn't lie, and it is contagious. The people we share space with and the environments we find ourselves in directly impact our nervous systems. Sensory language is just as powerful as words because the goodness, sweetness, and delight linger.

Empathy is one of the gifts that naturally comes with protecting our energy because we have an increased capacity to hold space for others, which in turn increases our sense of connection. When we tend to and take care of our energy, it grows and is palpable in our relationships. It helps us soften into compassion and kindness, model regulation and flexibility, and uplift those we love, which is all needed now more than ever in the world. Our abundant, overflowing energy helps us show up with our whole selves and awaken to the injustices around us, leading to both self and community healing.

Our embodiment practices are political, and they give us more fuel for the fight ahead, especially in the political landscape we are currently navigating. Oppressive systems want us burnt out and exhausted because that gives them more control. Your sensitivity and rage are both needed, and tending to your nervous system amid it all is a sacred act. I wonder what could happen if we looked at our ability to feel so deeply when we witness heartbreaking events in the world as a sign of our humanity and the depth of our hearts. In a world that is often numb to the pain and suffering of others, your ability to care deeply is a gift. Meeting this moment in history means remembering that caring for each other is all we have.

When well-balanced with strong boundaries, empathy is an essential component of the human experience that allows us to build trust, warmth, and generosity with others as we navigate the world. But it can be hard to access it when we are feeling run down. I know there are times when my empathy meter was in the red because I hadn't taken the time to care for myself. This, of course, directly impacted my ability and capacity to hold space and demonstrate my care for loved ones, which never feels good.

In their book *Sensitive*, the authors Jenn Granneman and Andre Sólo share that when we are able to respond with warmth to someone else's suffering, it actually changes our brain chemistry. When we have the capacity to express compassion (a close companion to empathy), "our heart rate slows, we release the 'bonding hormone' oxytocin, and the parts of the brain linked to caregiving and pleasure light up."[4] We, of course, don't want to give away all of ourselves to the point when we have nothing left, but one of the perks of tending to our energy is the ability to prioritize creating more space in our lives so all those worthy of our care and attention can access it when needed. **Offering your care while simultaneously being grounded in your boundaries is a generous act.**

As we will continue to explore together, self-care and community care are interconnected. Prioritizing our own energy is one of the key ways to help us build our empathy and compassion reservoirs, so let's unpack how we can be more intentional about this process.

Taking Stock of the Ebbs and Flows of Your Energy

Now that we have a clear understanding of why it's important to protect our energy, let's delve into the various ways we can get practical about assessing it. By bringing awareness to the various ways our energy is drained throughout the day, we can find clarity (and grace) when beginning to identify the practices that can help life become not just more manageable but more fulfilling.

One of the practices that helped me make immediate shifts in my life is the somatic practice of *portioning*.[5] It first involves getting a sense of your current energy levels and bandwidth: How full or depleted do you feel in this moment? Take a moment right now to reflect on this question with the full senses of your mind, body, and spirit to assess your capacity and how much you have to give. Then take inventory of your schedule for the upcoming week—the activities, meetings, appointments, and anything else on your list that may require a large energetic output. See what can be moved around, canceled, or otherwise adjusted to help you increase your margins. This is the portioning part of the practice—making space, delegating, and putting buffers in place to keep you from unintentionally draining your energy.

Another practice that has worked wonders in my life is setting time aside for micro-moments of self-care and rest. In these spaces, I soften my gaze or lie down for as many minutes as I can grab throughout the day. This might seem like a simple practice, but it is not always intuitive, as many of us have become accustomed to mindlessly and quickly moving through our schedule and tasks instead of resting. This small exercise has the potential to bring awareness to your unchecked aversions to rest and help you identify where you can start creating more space for yourself. It also allows for much-needed breaks from the constant overstimulation that drains your energy. Whether we realize it or not, many of us have been conditioned to view rest as lazy, unproductive behavior, but this only causes us more distress in the long run. In her book *The Relaxed Woman*, Nicola Jane Hobbs shares, "Each time I work through lunch or trade sleep for productivity or reply to an email outside of work hours, I'm normalizing these things. Each time I push through when I'm exhausted, I'm contributing to societal expectations that [others] do the same. Each time I judge my worth by how much I get done in a day, I'm contributing to a culture of toxic productivity."[6] When we can instead prioritize more restful and compassionate ways of being, through our own modeling and boundaries, we start to normalize this behavior through a positive lens.

In my workshops and classes, I frequently pose the gentle inquiry: How often do you find yourself replicating the urgency and frenetic pace of your life on your yoga mat? We often unintentionally create this parallel process, but we are worthy of taking off our armor and resting in ways that feel safe, *especially* on our yoga mat. We don't have to continue to succumb to grind culture in spaces designed for us to decompress. In the moments when it all feels so hard (even resting), remember that deprograming from the harmful impacts of toxic capitalism and urgency culture takes not just awareness of the gravity of all we have carried but also time.

We are constantly navigating messages that we need to just push through. We deserve space in our lives to *just be*. Our nervous systems need an abundance of rest to thrive. In order to do this, we have to take stock of the small choices we might be making each and every day that negatively affect our energy and time. These are the micro-moments that accumulate into chronic feelings of exhaustion and stress. I invite you to read the following statements and take note of which, if any, sound familiar to you:

- I'm just going to respond to this email real quick.
- Let me just send this document before we go.
- I am going to try to squeeze this appointment into my schedule.
- I have to fill out this school form.
- I just need to pay this bill real quick.
- I need to call them back right now.
- I need to get gas and squeeze in an oil change before my meeting.
- I have to fit in a grocery store trip and errands today.
- The laundry is stressing me out, and I can't relax until it's done and put away.
- The trash can is overflowing, and I need to take it out before we go.
- I am so behind on my texts.
- The house is so dirty, and I am overstimulated by it all.
- I need to drop off these returns today.
- I need to research that program/activity for the kids.
- I need to meal prep this week.
- We have to finish homework quickly before we go to soccer.
- I missed my dentist appointment and need to pay the late fee and reschedule.
- Let me RSVP to this before I forget.

I know how all-encompassing the "admin of life" can be, and I know how the pressure to pick up the phone or finish that task is like a magnet that pulls us in. And I certainly do not want to minimize the very real impact of the mental load we carry daily or the tasks that must get done to keep everything running smoothly. I find myself in this struggle constantly. To be honest, there is always going to be someone who is waiting on a response from us, and there is always going to be something else on our lists that needs our attention. We have been so deeply programmed to give in to these cycles of urgency that even when we have a minute to sit down and be, our mind starts tracking to the next task, convincing us that it absolutely has to be done at this very moment—or else!

You may think it's no big deal to quickly respond to emails or complete tasks during every waking moment, but I invite you to consider the impact of these seemingly small choices that chip into your energy. This accumulation of "just one more thing" is one of the many reasons deep exhaustion feels so pervasive; many of us are operating from a "chronic rest deficit."[7] You do not need to be productive every minute of your life. In fact, that is the very mindset that is keeping you stuck in cycles of exhaustion. (More on this when we discuss the intentional practice of rest in chapter 6.)

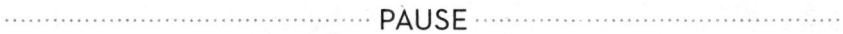

PAUSE

A Nourishing Practice to Soften the Overwhelm

This is a moment to pause and explore a nourishing practice to help soften your overwhelm with love and care. For this practice, I invite you to explore the various ways you can activate your parasympathetic nervous system and find a deep sense of embodied restoration. Take as much time as you need to set up for your practice in a way that supports a sense of ease and peace and allows you to gently tune out the outside world and tune in to your needs. If it feels supportive, you might rest a heavy blanket over your body, draw a bolster or a pillow underneath your knees for added support, or roll up some blankets and allow your arms to rest on them. Any prop or position that allows you to feel lifted, held, and supported is perfect.

Once you're settled in your space, take a deep, full inhale, then exhale and allow everything to soften. If it feels right, you can rest a palm on your heart and a palm on your belly and take note of the rise and fall of your beautiful, powerful breath. Allow the power of your breath to serve as an anchor throughout this practice, something you can come back to when the thoughts start to swirl, when your to-do list starts to creep in.

Soften your breath to the degree that feels right and safe for you. For a moment, can you take all of that compassion that you pour out into everything and everyone and pour it back into yourself? Can you breathe in your own light, your own energy, your own affection, your own support? For a moment, within the container of this space, can you take everything that you've been carrying and holding within and let it roll off of your shoulders and onto the support that holds you here? Can you let yourself feel held? Can you remind yourself that you are never alone in your experience?

Now gently inhale and explore an open-mouth exhale. Can you let the strength of your body meet the power of your breath? When you feel ready, and if you're able, I invite you into Adi Mudra. Draw your thumbs into your palms and then wrap your fingers around your thumbs like you're making a fist. If this is not possible for you, you can rest your hands in any way that feels good, palms facing toward the sky or down toward the ground.

In Adi Mudra, you are always in control of how much you'd like to squeeze your thumbs. Maybe start to modulate here and see what feels best for you. Allow your shoulders to relax up, back, and down your spine and take a moment to allow your breath to ground you. All of these actions are working to ease your overwhelm and help you delegate, ask for help, or *do something just for you.*

Continue breathing at your pace. If you'd like, you can cross your arms across your chest, coming into a butterfly hug, and offer yourself your own care. You might gently rock side to side here. If it feels okay, you can even rest your cheek on top of your palm. Take a moment here to invite in a little compassion, a little ease, a little tenderness, a little softness. Continue like this for as long as it feels good.

Coming back to center, bring your palms to the back of your shoulders if you're able and give yourself a gentle self-massage. Take note of any parts of your being that might be holding constriction or tension. All of your parts are deserving of care and tenderness. If you'd like, you can continue the self-massage on the back of your head, on your temples, down your forearms, or on the soles of your feet. Continue to invite in that deep sense of rest and nurturing support. Take all the time you need, beloved; there's absolutely no rush.

When you feel ready, and only if it feels supportive, I invite you to come into a supported Bridge Pose (Setu Bandhasana). If this does not feel right for you, stay exactly as you are. To ease into this posture, you are welcome to rest on your back, drawing the soles of your feet to the mat or ground underneath you and resting your arms by your side. On your inhale, lift up your hips and gently slide a block or another support underneath your lower back if needed. On your exhale, melt your sacrum (or tailbone) into the block, finding that sweet spot and feeling that sense of support. Make any adjustments to increase your comfort. Stay here for a few moments, listening to the sound of your breath. Start to slow everything down. You are worthy of receiving this support.

When you feel ready, on your inhale, lift your hips up and release the block. In your own time and in your own way, find a comfortable seated position, bringing in any movement that feels right for you. Maybe you feel inclined to wiggle your fingers and toes or circle your wrists and ankles. You could interlace your palms overhead and lengthen your spine all the way up to the crown of your head. Perhaps a few neck rolls or half circles feel good. Do whatever feels most accessible to you.

Once you've welcomed some movement back into your body, place your palms at the center of your heart or find any other expression that aligns with a sense of gratitude. Hands at your heart, may we live our lives compassionately. Hands at your mouth, may we speak words of truth and kindness. And hands at your third-eye center, the light in me always honors the light in you.

I encourage you to take this rested, gentle, compassionate energy with you into the rest of your day. You deserve this feeling of peace and ease.

To access an audio recording of this meditation,
visit us.macmillan.com/ProtectYourEnergy.

....

Assessing Your Energy

If you were to take a scan of what a typical day looks like for you, where do *you* fit in? Not the things you are constantly doing for others but the time that is designated to nurturing you and you alone. I invite you to reflect on the following questions in your journal to help you take note of where your energy is being chipped away and how to begin reclaiming it. There is no need to assign numbers, metrics, or judgments to your responses. This is a space for you to gently sit with your answers and build awareness around how you can start protecting your energy. So, grab your journal, take your time to jot down whatever wants to be explored, and as always *be so very gentle.*

PHYSICAL

- When you feel irritability and resentment arise, where do you feel it in your body?
- Do you take your full lunch breaks (perhaps not in front of a screen) to restore and recalibrate?
- Do you prioritize moving your body in ways that bring you joy? Or does there never feel like there is enough time?
- Are you able to integrate moments of rest and downregulation throughout the day, or do you find that your activities run back to back?
- Do you prioritize your health and regularly attend doctor's appointments (dentist, general physician, therapy, holistic healing support, specialists)?

EMOTIONAL

- When you receive a triggering or activating email, do you respond right away?
- Do you have any outlets (therapist, healers, support system, community) to help you process the depth of what you might be holding?

- Are you able to integrate or prioritize play into your life? Why or why not?
- When you do have time to decompress at the end of your day, are you able to enjoy it and be present with your family or yourself?
- Are you able to pause, reflect, and celebrate all that it's taken to get to this point in your life and remember that it is beautiful and enough? Or do you find yourself constantly focusing on "What's next?"

MENTAL

- When you have space on your calendar, do you protect it? Or can you be convinced to schedule over time dedicated for yourself?
- What's your process for asking for help when you are overwhelmed?
- How would you describe your relationship with your boundaries? Are you able to stick to them, or do you tend to bend or work around them?
- Do you read books that are non–self-help related?
- Do you protect the time you've designated for certain projects, or do you find yourself consistently getting distracted by the "urgent" needs of others throughout the day?
- Do you consistently work late into the evening?

SPIRITUAL

- What is the first thing you do when you wake up in the morning?
- Are you able to create space for spiritual practices, routines, or sacred rituals that are meaningful or fulfilling to you? What does this mean for you?
- How would you describe the quality of your day?
- When you think about your life holistically, what does success mean to you? And if you could redefine what success looks like, how would it look?
- How do you connect to your sense of community and purpose?

These questions may seem simple, but they are a powerful and revealing way to begin to assess how you expend your energy. From here, we will continue the deeper work of swapping out depleting habits for more restorative ones.

The Dimensions of Energy

There are a number of ways for us to be in relationship with our energy. As you begin to assess your energy expenditure, I invite you to identify the things that are currently draining you within the different energy dimensions you just explored—physical, emotional, mental, and spiritual. Feel free to look back to your journaling session to help guide this process.

For example, if you are mentally drained, this might mean that your brain is completely full with the mental load you have been carrying—life admin, caregiving responsibilities, work tasks, family and social obligations. Even if you delegate, you may not feel any relief because you continue to worry about whether or not the task is going to get done or if it'll be done well. You have trouble fully releasing it, not just from your list but also from your mind and body. If you are emotionally drained, it may mean that you have been absorbing the stressors and struggles of others in addition to dealing with your own. Perhaps you haven't found the proper outlets to process it all.

If you are physically drained, you might be simply pushing yourself too hard in all areas of your life—working long hours, doing strenuous workouts, saying yes to every request, and so forth. Existing in these states of depletion is when rest might feel more like collapse than restoration. If you are spiritually drained, it might mean you have moved further and further away from the places, people, and activities that renew and replenish your spirit and light you up. Perhaps you have been grinding every day and spending less time connected to nature or practices where you find that deep sense of awe, belonging, creativity, and purpose that bring your nervous system a sense of ease. Setting and implementing embodied boundaries are foundational to each of these dimensions, which we will define more fully and explore in chapter 4.

I invite you to cultivate an intimate connection with these different dimensions of energy and take small steps each day to begin the important internal work of getting honest with yourself about where you are feeling most drained. Bringing awareness to this aspect of your life can be hard and vulnerable, yet it can also be empowering to have a clear picture of where your energy is going and get to the root of your depletion.

When I became aware of the various aspects of my life that were leading to my depletion, it finally started to feel like something I could begin to tackle. It gave me a sense of control. We all need our own unique road map to reconnect to our spirit when we have drifted away from ourselves. In this process of self-discovery, you'll likely also end up highlighting the unmet needs you have, such as wanting to feel seen and supported with the mental load, receiving mental health support, and having time for "self-preservation" activities such as regular exercise, engaging with community, and spending time in nature. But being able to identify where you need more space and support is the first step, beloved.

What did you notice in your body as you reflected on your energy drains in the previous journaling exercise? Can you gently bring awareness to the parts of your body that might be holding tension, feeling constricted, or experiencing blocks where your nervous system is craving flow? Spend some time journaling what it would look like if you paid more attention to the areas of your life where your energy is being drained and started to take tangible steps toward protecting it.

Energy Protection Practices

Be more generous, kind, and gentle with yourself, beloved.

In this next section, I offer a number of energy protection practices. Continue to build upon your journaling by taking note of the practices here that feel the most accessible for you. These are just a few ideas, so I invite you to make note of the ones that resonate with you and tailor them to your unique situation. Protecting your energy is an everyday intentional practice, and you are worthy of building daily rituals that support filling your cup instead of draining it.

TENDING TO AND REPLENISHING YOUR MENTAL ENERGY

- **Check in with yourself before checking in with the world.** When we first wake in the morning, we often allow the outside world to dictate our mood before our bodies are even fully awake. This is the quickest way to activate the sympathetic nervous system and throw off your day. Taking the time to check in with yourself each morning can be just what you need to start off your day on the right foot. It doesn't need to be anything fancy; simple activities such as stretching, writing, or breathing can be enough to grant you a few sacred moments to start your day (think preventative self-care).

  Your email inbox, social media, responsibilities, and family will all be awaiting you, but that morning check-in can help you tend to and nurture your spirit. Over time and with repetition, this can have a profound impact on the quality of your energy as you move throughout your day.

- **Revise your to-do list as the day goes on.** Instead of trying to rush and tackle five things on your list, try to do just one very well. Practice intention by not running that extra errand, squeezing in that outing, or doing anything to overextend yourself (especially when the day is already full and bursting). Make it a habit to check in with your internal energy meter as you move through your day, and whenever possible, let that take precedence over your to-do list.

- **Take in less information and apply what you already know.** I love this reminder because in the age of information overload, we can easily trick ourselves into believing we don't have enough information to make a decision or even begin our healing process. This can leave us in a state of constant striving as we grasp for more answers. Start with where you are and what you know. Your body is wise. Let it be a guide to help you navigate everyday choices and challenges.

- **Take your full lunch break, not in front of a screen.** This is one of the most significant energy depleters I see in professionals who often multitask during the only planned break they have during the day. Offer yourself grace and be unapologetic about reclaiming this time for yourself.
- **Practice moving slower.** Slowing down is one of the key pathways to healing the nervous system. Take note of the moments you are rushing in your day and mindfully practice turning it down a few notches (when you are brushing your teeth, eating, driving somewhere, doing the dishes, etc.). Start to notice the subtle shifts that come about from doing daily tasks a little more slowly.
- **Acknowledge the systems of oppression that create barriers instead of unfairly blaming yourself.** In the introduction we explored some forms of systemic oppression that add to the layers of exhaustion historically marginalized folks experience on a daily basis. If you find yourself exhausted by these things, please know that your exhaustion is seen and so deeply valid, and it is not your fault. We are worthy of finding ways to meet the resistance by tending to ourselves and our experiences with compassion and care. We all deserve more support and resources to manage simply being human. Gently releasing yourself from the shame you might be experiencing from "not being able to do it all" and acknowledging the things that are outside of your control can offer you moments of self-compassion in the larger framework of your life.
- **Be mindful of trauma consumption.** Especially if you have a highly sensitive nervous system, be mindful of how often you consume traumatic news stories, movies, shows, social media posts, books, podcasts, and even conversations with friends. Trauma consumption is a subtle form of energetic depletion that can accumulate and compound the other challenges you may be managing in your life.

- **Indulge in the small things.** Don't underestimate the power of a solo drive, an amazing playlist, a delicious coffee, fresh sheets, a nourishing meal, less stimulation, an easeful morning, a clear schedule, a hug, the support of a friend or loved one, a dance party, the sunset, and sleep. All of these things have the ability to chip away at your overwhelm and help turn your day around. Find the glimmers in these moments.

TENDING TO AND REPLENISHING YOUR EMOTIONAL ENERGY

- **Offer yourself the gift of self-compassion.** Practice repeating the following phrases to show yourself some compassion and grace:
  - *I am so proud of how I am navigating this.*
  - *It is completely understandable that I am this overwhelmed. I can make a new plan that honors my current capacity. I don't have to overextend myself.*
  - *So many people feel this way too. I am not alone in my experience.*
  - *I am feeling anxious in this moment, but it is not my whole identity.*
  - *I am doing my best, and that is always enough.*
  - *I don't have to power through this. It all can wait. I can rest.*
  - *Just because someone is disappointed with my boundary does not mean I need to change it or do anything that brings me discomfort or unease.*
  - *It doesn't have to be perfect. I can give myself grace.*
  - *I can take my time. I don't have to rush my process.*
  - *I am worthy of my own love, respect, and care. I can make choices that reflect that knowing.*
- **Create a resourcing corner.** Create a sanctuary space or corner in your home that is just for you and for the sake of energy preservation, pause, and stillness. Choose a place you can return to regularly that brings you ease and comfort. Don't skimp on anything that feels supportive or indulgent.

Think comfy blankets and socks, a cozy beanbag seat, your favorite journal, eye pillows, candles, or your own version of ease and comfort.

- **Remember to remember yourself.** Life can get hard, intense, and full. In a society that expects persistent busyness, we are often bound by schedules, an unsustainable pace, and constant cycles of overwhelm. It is no wonder that when we finally slow down and release the distractions, unresolved emotions often make their way to the surface. Our emotions are information, and there is so much that can get locked inside when we constantly keep ourselves busy with external factors.

  So, what does it look like to be more generous and kind to yourself? I often have to say to myself, *Remember to remember yourself.* This simple phrase helps bring me back to the present moment and the parts of me that need playfulness, joy, freedom, and space to just be.

- **Be mindful of the energy you let in.** You are one person in a great big world with things constantly vying for your attention and time. Not everything or every emotion is yours to carry. You are doing your best, and that will always be enough. Perhaps there are triggering social media accounts that you can block or mute, times you can put your phone on Do Not Disturb, space where you can notice when you feel overwhelmed, boundaries you can set with people who drain your energy, or environments and people you can be unapologetic about surrounding yourself with. Everything you consume and engage with can impact your nervous system, so as best as you can, be intentional with what you allow in your space.

- **Nurture relationships with people who are good for your nervous system.** Have you ever left an interaction with someone knowing deep down that they were good for your well-being? As best as you can, prioritize nurturing those relationships, even in small ways like with text messages, handwritten letters, or coffee dates. You deserve that good energy in your life.

- **Tangible support can renew your spirit.** The psychotherapist Katherine Morgan Schafler calls tangible support "practical aid."[8] This is the kind of support that directly benefits your daily life and takes a load off your shoulders, such as a loved one coming over to help you clean your house, drop off food, or spend time with your child while you sleep or complete a task. During some of my darkest days, just brushing my teeth and washing my face was a monumental task. I couldn't even fathom doing anything beyond that as the grief completely overwhelmed my nervous system. It was this kind of tangible and practical support, love, and compassion from my community that kept me floating on that life raft. Asking for and receiving help can offer the most sacred form of energy restoration.

TENDING TO AND REPLENISHING YOUR PHYSICAL ENERGY

- **Portion your energy output.** The somatic practice we completed earlier known as *portioning* invites you to take stock of how full or depleted an average week makes you feel and make mindful changes in your schedule moving forward to preserve your energy. Similarly, this practice invites you to make note of what events, activities, or tasks can be moved, delegated, or canceled altogether to make space for restorative time. This new awareness around your schedule has the ability to have a profound impact on how you steward your energy and care.
- **Take a restorative yoga class instead of always opting for a rigorous one.** So often when we are trying to squeeze in exercise or movement of any kind, we put a lot of pressure on ourselves to "make the most of it" and choose something high energy or intense. Of course there is nothing wrong with this, but every once in a while, I invite you to take stock of what your body is holding, the kind of week you have had, and the challenges you are currently navigating and pay attention to the type of practice your body may

be craving. We can deplete our energy reserves even more when we push our bodies during workouts instead of giving into rest.

- **Give yourself the gift of more rest.** Our nervous systems benefit from an overflow of rest. Please be gentle with yourself when you realize that you might need more recovery time than others. Trust and honor your unique ecosystem and lived experience and give your body the gift of replenishment for all it does for you. Pace yourself and focus on attuning to your needs, moment to moment.
- **Listen to the cues of your nervous system.** Can you pause and give yourself what you need as soon as you recognize those first warning signals of exhaustion? Tending to your needs as soon as you become aware of them allows you to preserve and protect your bandwidth not only in the moment but for tomorrow as well. The daily choices you make to prioritize the health of your nervous system help you slowly build toward the overflow. Be patient with yourself, love.

TENDING TO AND REPLENISHING YOUR SPIRITUAL ENERGY

- **Clean up the mess a little at a time.** I imagine many of us can relate to the sheer overwhelm of taking a look at our space and feeling like our whole lives are out of control. The clinical psychologist Becky Kennedy has a mantra that often rings true in my mind: "The house is a mess, but I am not a mess."[9] Give yourself grace and practice cleaning up the mess a little at a time. Start with just one thing. One dish. One piece of clothing in the drawer. One toy. One text. One email. One boundary. Whatever your "one" thing is, celebrate the small wins.
- **Have a plan for dealing with people who drain your spirit.** Try to prepare in advance before entering interactions with people you know drain your energy. Set boundaries around how much time you will spend with them, prepare

to pause a conversation if you feel your sympathetic nervous system being activated, give yourself permission to take breaks or have a plan to leave, or practice the energy protection meditation in chapter 6 beforehand.

- **Protect your self-replenishment time.** This is truly where all the magic happens. Once this becomes a daily, embodied ritual, no matter how short or long, you begin to build neuroplasticity and honoring yourself becomes nonnegotiable.

- **If possible, try to resist the urge to fill the space.** When you have been accustomed to living in survival mode for so long, it's normal to feel the urge to fill up any free time or pauses in your day. Instead, try to savor these in-between moments. Dedicate them to yourself and carve out rituals of care. You deserve to know what slowing down actually feels like.

- **Practice spiritual hygiene.** Throughout each day, the various interactions and energies you encounter can essentially "stick" to you and have an influence on your mood and energy levels. This is why it's important to implement rituals throughout your day to cleanse your spirit of anything that feels particularly charged or activating. Some examples might include dancing, walking, journaling, praying, or any tangible rituals that allow you to energetically transition from one person or part of your day to the next.

- **Resource yourself.** Resourcing is the act of mindfully identifying a person, place, sound, or thing that generates feelings of well-being, neutrality, peace, comfort, joy, or calm to bring you out of an activated state. Perhaps this could be a good friend, an emotional support pet, your favorite song, or even a quiet place out in nature. Once you become aware of what resources bring you peace, you can come back to them throughout the day when your energy needs a boost.

- **Practice an embodied check-in before taking on additional commitments.** Before you take on that new project or client, check in with yourself and your current capacity. Is it something that can be delayed to give yourself space? Do you actually need to say yes in this moment? What cues do you receive from your body when you envision taking this on? Trust your body's responses to your inquiries and move accordingly.

GENTLE REMINDER

You deserve more than perpetual states of burnout and taking on more at the expense of your health.

Replenishing and Protecting Your Energy

Now that you are aware of the energy-replenishing practices that are available to you, take a moment in your journal to identify which ones you'd like to implement in your life in each energy dimension. Please don't put pressure on yourself to fill each category with a number of to-dos. **The act of caring for yourself does not need to be another stressful thing on your list.** There is nothing to prove and no one to impress. Take your time and be gentle with yourself.

Each day, we are exposed to a lot of external pressure to try to keep all the balls afloat, but less is more when it comes to a nervous-system-informed framework. This journey involves paying close attention to your current needs and capacity and what your body is communicating to you (choosing to stretch instead of doing a strenuous workout, picking a family-friendly activity that does not require a large energetic output, allowing yourself to take breaks from work and daily life, etc.). This is not something you need to rush, excel in, or perfect. In fact, part of the process is taking missteps, scanning your days, and allowing your light and energy to become your main priority.

Give yourself permission to not overachieve at this. You might focus on just one dimension of energy that needs your attention, or perhaps you'll commit to the practices and frameworks of care that excite and revive you and that, most importantly, *feel manageable*. Pick the starting points that make sense for you and feel seamless in bringing you a deep sense of ease.

In his *New York Times* bestselling book *Atomic Habits*, the author James Clear reminds us of the power of "making small improvements on a daily basis" and how "too often we convince ourselves that massive success requires massive action." His entire framework speaks to the power of small, digestible steps and how the impact over time can be astounding.[10] I invite you to apply this approach to all the ways you nurture your mental, physical, emotional, and spiritual energy. Keep showing up for yourself daily, no matter how small it feels, and take stock of the cumulative shifts you begin to notice in your life over time.

I encourage you to take a moment to explore the Assessing Your Energy worksheet, available in the "Additional Resources" section of the book, for a tangible tool to check in with your energy and capacity. Bookmark this resource anytime you need gentle guidance for getting honest about your needs, checking back in with yourself, and coming back to your center.

I hope this chapter has helped you become aware of the fact that there are so many micro-moments within the context of your day that can chip away at your energy. When you really start to pause and conceptualize the cumulative impact that this has on your nervous system, it can be incredibly eye-opening. We can get so caught up in the constant need to stay in motion and overgive and overwork (often as an escape from our feelings). Sometimes we need the gentle reminder that no amount of tasks can take away our enoughness and wholeness. Our gifts are deeply inherent, not something we need to strive for or achieve. We can honor what needs tending to in each season, ask for what we need, and remember that we are worthy of centering our humanity as we navigate the often relentless pace of our lives.

In the next chapter, we will get a little more honest with ourselves as we begin to examine all the ways we push through and beyond our limits. When we try to function without boundaries around our time, energy, capacity, and spirit, things can start to fall apart because we rarely give ourselves space for restoration. Instead, our time is frequently filled with giving and being of service to others. What if we could reconceptualize a new, softer way? One that allowed more room for grace, ease, self-prioritization, and nourishing practices? Let's explore the possibilities together.

3

You Can't—and Shouldn't—Do It All

One of the most loving things you can do for yourself is to give yourself permission to not always have your shit together. This life will constantly oscillate between seasons of order and disorder. The question is: can you still love yourself when your mess is showing?[1]
—JONATHAN LOUIS DENT

Years ago, I was attending a workshop where the facilitators distributed a "self-care assessment checklist." We were instructed to go down the list and number on a scale of one to five how well or not well we do certain things related to self-care. There was one in particular that stopped me in my tracks: "How often do you allow yourself to *not* be the one leading all of the time or in charge of something?" I could think of countless examples where I did just the opposite, and it made me think of the various roles I have carried, all the times I didn't delegate or ask for help when I desperately needed to, and how often I "pushed through" and did it all on my own. I honestly got emotional thinking about how much of my life I had spent feeling overwhelmed.

I immediately got on the phone with my therapist to tell her about my new revelation. She said, "Zabie, have you ever in your life just thought to yourself, *So what if I don't do this thing, if this person is disappointed by my boundary, if I just let this thing go, etc.?*"

I released my shoulders from the tops of my ears and said, "Absolutely not." I had spent so much time managing the emotional roller coaster of fearing other people's disappointment. Over time, I have come to learn that this stems from my tendency to overgive.

With the utmost intention, care, and power, consider this chapter your permission to stop overextending yourself. As much as we may want to believe the contrary, overextending ourselves does *not* make people respect us more. In fact, if you keep giving, people will just keep taking. The hard truth is, as the author and wellness educator Alex Elle reminds us, "You will encounter some people in this life who you will never be enough for. No matter how good you are, no matter how loving you are, no matter how intentional you are. You cannot keep running yourself ragged."[2]

Where can you create a little more space in your life for your mind, body, and spirit to rest? Where can you delegate some tasks to others, ask for help, or begin to set boundaries with how you want to expend your energy? As often as you can, send an abundance of compassion to the many versions of you that have made it to this point in your life. Those versions were needed to get you to the level of awareness you now have in this moment. As you continue through this chapter, my hope is that you realize that sometimes the most powerful embodiment practice is learning how to do *less* instead of always doing more.

Productivity Does Not Equal Worthiness

In her book *I Didn't Do the Thing Today*, the researcher Madeleine Dore reminds us of the dangers of conflating productivity with worthiness. "There's the laundry thing, the catch-up thing, the replying to a text thing, the grocery shopping thing, the work thing, the medical thing, the thing we ought to do, the thing we don't want to do, the thing we've put off despite it being the one important thing."[3] When all of these things become urgent, our nervous systems can start to become hijacked by even seemingly small stressors. We can become so accustomed to overstimulation and programmed for chaos that learning how to be still and find much-needed spaciousness can be incredibly challenging and even unsettling at times.

As I shared earlier, I find that so much of my work these days is supporting folks in exploring what it means to rest in ways that feel safe for them. Often this practice can be a catalyst for them to begin weaving daily decompression of the nervous system into the fabric of their everyday lives. I want to let you know that you, too, are worthy of exploring what this looks like for you at your pace and in your time. The power lies in your embodied boundaries and your commitment and accountability to yourself.

If you're like me, you may need some tangible examples of what it might look like to no longer overextend yourself, so take a look at the following list and consider which of these you'd be open to implementing in your life:

- Releasing and softening the juggling act and perpetual cycles of burnout
- Evaluating what is on your plate and getting honest with yourself about what can be released (e.g., not sending holiday cards, not enrolling your child in another extracurricular activity, or resisting the urge to go above and beyond)
- Replacing your quick yes with "I need time to think about that request"
- Responding to requests at your pace instead of getting caught up in other people's urgency
- Delegating tasks to others or letting someone else volunteer
- Being clear and kind with your wants and needs
- Trusting what you need and listening to your inner voice
- Canceling or rescheduling when you need time for yourself
- Not doing that thing (yes, *that* one)
- Offering yourself more grace and less pressure
- Giving yourself time in your day to just sit and be
- Letting yourself enjoy slowness and stillness and feeling your exhale

A Nervous System Reset for All Who Are Overextended

This practice offers you an opportunity to reconnect with your nervous system in a restorative way if you are feeling burnt out and overscheduled. Taking the time to intentionally slow down, honor your body's messages, and respond in ways that feel kind and compassionate is an integral part of the healing journey.

I invite you to take a moment to rub your palms together to create a little bit of warmth, and then gently rest them on any parts of the body that feel exhausted, depleted, or worn out. Where do you feel that showing up in your body? You might rest them over your eyes to soothe sensory stimulation and tend to the mental load. You may gently massage your temples, the backs of your shoulders, your forearms, your palms, or any other parts of your body that feel the weight of all you have carried. You might even wrap your arms around your body for a nourishing hug to take in your own care.

If you would like, explore interlacing your fingers and bringing your palms to the back of your head for a gentle cradle. Breathe into your light, breathe into your heart. Inhale to shine your heart and draw your energy up toward the sky, and exhale to draw everything inward by bringing your elbows toward your body. You might repeat this a few times, connecting your breath to your movement. If it feels right, you might rest your right palm on your right cheek for a compassionate face cradle. Hold yourself in all of the care and tenderness. Switch sides whenever you feel ready. You might explore rubbing your palms back together to come back to your inner light and then rest both palms over your heart.

I encourage you to offer yourself this kind of self-compassion and gentleness any time you are feeling overextended or overwhelmed. There's always time to engage in a brief moment of self-care.

To access an audio recording of this meditation,
visit us.macmillan.com/ProtectYourEnergy.

Holding the Default Nervous System in the Room

When I learned the term *default nervous system*,[4] it helped me name my ongoing struggle: always being on and feeling the constant pressure to have a regulated and flexible nervous system in order to provide a sense of safety and co-regulation for all those I typically hold space for. In essence, I found that I was the emotional regulator that everyone leaned on. Whether in parenting, caregiving, leading, teaching, running a business, space holding, or simply showing up daily as we tend to our own wounds, so many of us can relate to always holding the default nervous system in the room.

One moment you might be crying in your car as you contend with your inner world, and five minutes later you might be leading a staff meeting where everyone is looking to you to fulfill their requests and manage their grievances. This could also look like waking up in the morning after a challenging night's sleep to tiny humans waiting for you to meet their every need. Even on the days we may not be dealing with something particularly heavy, we may still feel the pressure to always hold it together and be a grounding presence. When we hold the default nervous system in the room in this way, others often "borrow" from our nervous system to support their own. That is a huge responsibility and a lot of pressure any way you slice it.

I don't think we talk enough about how hard this is and the longing many of us have to feel seen through it all. Sometimes with the little energy we have left, we simply do not have the bandwidth to explain how much we may be struggling. But we are worthy of being able to turn our brains off or at least turn the volume down. I also think when we recognize our weariness in these moments and try to tend to our basic needs, we can sometimes deprive ourselves of the totality or fullness of the experience. I attribute much of this to urgency culture because many of us are wired to *do* and *respond* before we are actually ready to. For example, Jennifer Cohen Harper, a trauma-sensitive mindfulness educator and author, asked caregivers how often they say things like "I'm just going to take a quick shower," "I'm going to grab a quick bite to eat," or "I'm running to the bathroom real quick" as a buffer to those in our environment.[5] Phew, I have certainly said some variation of these things many times.

I can think of countless times I have said to my husband, "I am going to squeeze in a quick workout" or "I will be ready in five minutes!" With this observation, Cohen Harper sheds light on how important it is to "meet our human needs without rushing." What if, instead, you practiced doing these things *real slowly*? Next time you feel inclined to rush through what your heart needs in the moment, take some time to pause and remember that you are worthy of your own time and attention. Even when the house is a mess. Even when there are beloveds waiting on you. Even when there are pending items on your to-do list. Even when the emails and texts keep pinging. You are your most precious resource, and you deserve to honor yourself through that lens and mindfully take the time you need.

Not feeling rushed is so deeply healing and perhaps a love language all on its own.

Not feeling rushed is so deeply healing and perhaps a love language all on its own.

Not feeling rushed is so deeply healing and perhaps a love language all on its own.

Not feeling rushed is so deeply healing and perhaps a love language all on its own.

The "Seemingly Small" Yeses

I frequently find myself staring out the window, reflecting on the cumulative impact of the "seemingly small" things we often say yes to. Whether it's a new project at work, additional caregiving tasks, or "just a tiny favor" for a friend, if you're anything like me, you likely find yourself saying yes to things when you'd really rather say no. Why is this?

Well, there are many reasons we may feel compelled to give in to others' requests when they very clearly go against what we might actually want to do in the moment. The discomfort of potentially disappointing others can be very loud. And when we are perpetually disconnected from our own needs, it can be very easy to continue to give *all* of ourselves away to others. Additionally, if we grew up learning that our own care is secondary to others, we may not even have the language to communicate what we are experiencing. There may also be scenarios we navigate at work or in caregiving where we feel like it is impossible to say no. This is one reason of many I feel passionate about the intersections between boundary work and nervous system work, which we will continue to explore in chapter 4. The more connected we are to ourselves, our needs, and our body cues, the more we can make informed decisions about where our energy goes.

Over the past several years, I have tried to honor myself and my capacity by practicing embodied check-ins before taking on more projects. (This was first introduced in the energy protection practices in chapter 2.) This doesn't have to be anything fancy, and it can be unique to you and the approach that feels most accessible. I've found the most peace in my life by pausing, resting a palm on my heart and my belly, gently connecting to the rise and fall of my breath, and sending love and tenderness to any parts of my body that feel exhausted, tense, or constricted. You may notice that I come back to this practice often in this book, and that's because it tends to offer people a powerful baseline of their capacity. Our bodies are always communicating with us; it's up to us to make time and space to listen.

Remember, the beauty of this healing journey is in its simplicity, so don't make a big fuss about coming up with the "perfect" embodied check-in. Some examples you can try might include slowing your pace, pausing to check in with yourself throughout the day, playing a restorative playlist, journaling about how it would *feel* in your body to take on a new project or task, or simply taking time to reflect before agreeing to a request. So often, just the awareness alone of pausing and *remembering to remember yourself* is a radical act that can help you create powerful shifts. In chapter 4 we will explore the somatics of boundaries and ask ourselves important questions (from a nervous system perspective) before we take on more.

> **GENTLE REMINDER**
>
> Our capacity is ongoing, fluid, and forever changing based on our current season of life. If you are navigating multiple stressors, your body might be craving more rest than usual. It's okay to honor the way your body is communicating to you instead of trying to intellectualize it or figure out why. And as the saying goes, it's okay to do less when you are dealing with more.

Your energy is sacred. You deserve the space to be thoughtful and intentional when making decisions that may bring you further or closer to yourself. Protecting your energy is such a radical practice because it allows you to bring awareness to the cumulative impact of both the small and large energy drains you may experience on any given day. You'll also be able to reconceptualize your needs in the larger framework of your life.

My energy is sacred.

My energy is sacred.

My energy is sacred.

My energy is sacred.

Humanizing and Exploring Your Needs and Care

Have you ever asked yourself what it would look like to get your needs met? Is this concept even on your radar? I imagine your needs list, like mine, is ongoing, ever-changing, and constantly evolving as you continue to heal and grow, so I encourage you to reflect on your needs often in your journal. Some of the things on my "needs" list include a slow, spacious schedule that allows me to take care of myself and tend to my daily responsibilities and, most importantly, help with the mental load.

The more tangible I can get with fulfilling my needs—putting the yoga class on my calendar, scheduling mental health days in advance as a preventative act of self-care, texting my partner a list of things I need help with, etc.—the more I'm able to feel like I have some semblance of control, and I can chip away at my exhaustion a little at a time. Part of this practice is knowing and believing that our hearts have the capacity to hold multiple truths at the same time. For example, it might be helpful to remember the following:

I CAN BE:	AND STILL:
resilient	need places where I can fall apart and not hold it all together
kind	set and honor boundaries that support my mental health
in love with my work	feel burnt out and need plenty of space for breaks and rest
committed to healing	need breaks from it all to thrive
a present and caring parent/caregiver	crave and seek out time alone
joyful	grieve

The board-certified psychiatrist Pooja Lakshmin defines "real self-care" as something that originates within us, an invisible and internal decision-making process that brings us closer to ourselves and our needs. It's about being intentionally aligned with our values, setting boundaries, moving past guilt, treating ourselves with compassion, meeting our needs, and taking up more space.[6] These descriptors feel so aligned with how I want to engage with my energy because they offer ways for us to come back to ourselves when the disconnection from our internal voice has become too strong.

My hope for all of us is that we celebrate this definition of self-care because it is a way to remember ourselves and our worth without the need to do more. Instead, it offers a gentle road map to help us feel empowered enough to slow down, process, and gain clarity around what feels most like *home*.

Getting My Needs Met Looks Like . . .

Although I have high ambitions for what it looks like to reclaim and protect my energy, I must be honest in saying that these days, getting my needs met is as simple as sitting in my car for ten minutes after my workday to listen to music, letting myself rest when I need to, and feeling the sun on my body. Other times, my needs feel larger, such as having a conversation with my partner about my current capacity ("I am running on fumes") and getting specific about what I need help with ("It would be a huge help to me if you could fill out this school form and enroll H in the soccer season").

My husband and I are typically very mindful about sharing the load in our home, but the truth is, in many partnerships, it is never going to be fifty-fifty. The scales are constantly tipping in one direction or the other because life, busy work seasons, stressors, unexpected challenges, triggers, and emotional overwhelm all constantly dip into our energy.

In a podcast episode with the entrepreneur and lifestyle coach Tim Ferriss, the researcher and motivational speaker Brené Brown shared a practice that she does with her partner where they intentionally and honestly share the percentage of their current capacity (10 percent, 25 percent, etc.). She says this allows them to be mindful of their energy levels and "figure out a plan of kindness toward each other."[7] I have found that building in buffers and margins like this as an ongoing practice to support the overall health and well-being of yourself and your loved ones is a deep practice of care.

Sometimes we may not even know how to articulate what we need because we are so used to powering through. But in particularly trying moments of life, even just articulating how we're feeling and getting support with the tangible tasks on our list is a form of protecting our precious and sacred energy. I know how deeply uncomfortable it can be for so many of us to ask for or receive help. We have gotten so used to managing on our own and doing things ourselves that we often say, "No, I'm fine, I got it!" when we could really benefit from the support. I was recently grocery shopping with my newborn and one of the Trader Joe's employees made eye contact with me and greeted me with such warmth and care. She insisted on grabbing my cart, walking around the store with me, and helping me get everything I needed. I felt so seen. I can only imagine if every caregiver had this type of support when they ventured out with a newborn! And honestly, my first inclination was to say, "No, it's okay. You don't have to do that!" But instead I leaned into the help and the support, which I needed more than I could express in that moment. So whether it is a seemingly small task or showing up for you in a larger way, the next time someone offers their assistance, I encourage you to practice accepting it. You deserve it.

I also invite you to spend some time considering the amount of space you allow yourself to take up in your own life. You may be used to prioritizing others. If so, putting your own care first for a change will require a radical and consistent reassessment and recalibration of what you need and how to achieve it so that you are not constantly operating from an empty well. I say radical because for many of us, this is not a comfortable process, nor is it something we tend to prioritize within the larger scope of our lives. You have to believe that you are worthy of deeply committing to yourself. I have goose bumps thinking of all the changes that await you, no matter how small they may feel at times. Magic lives there.

Self-Celebration and Validation
Right Here in the Middle

Getting comfortable with loving all parts of ourselves is a daily practice. Doing the internal work of protecting our energy and attuning to our embodied boundaries will not necessarily attract the external validation we may be seeking. We often celebrate others for their various achievements and milestones, but part of redefining what success looks like is learning to honor ourselves right here in the thick of our rebuilding process. In the thick of learning to take a pause before immediately saying yes, in the middle of setting boundaries regardless of others' disappointment, in the midst of starting to think about and prioritize our own feelings and needs instead of neglecting them and pushing through. These are all worthy of *so* much celebration!

We are quick to celebrate folks for doing the most, but our society is in desperate need of honoring and validating people for doing less. We typically save celebration for moments of "completion"—whatever that means—but we deserve celebration and acknowledgment right here in the middle.

On her podcast *The Deeper Call*, I shared with the author and somatic practitioner Ashley Neese about a miscarriage I had on New Year's Eve 2022.[8] The devastation of the loss was compounded by past experiences of trauma and also the starkness of what my family had envisioned for ourselves in the renewal and promise of a new year. I didn't have any intention of sharing that publicly at the time, but what unfolded in that conversation was the harsh truth that we often struggle silently in the moments we need the most support and encouragement. This moment of unexpected vulnerability inspired me to open up to my community as I moved through the process of fertility treatments instead of waiting until the outcome reached some point of closure that could be celebrated. This resulted in so many beloveds helping me put the pieces back together, offering priceless wisdom and love from their own experiences, holding space for the wide spectrum of triggers and emotions the process brought up, and holding my heart through an incredibly trying process that took so much out of me.

I didn't feel the need to mask the daily hardship, tears, and appointments I was enduring, and I felt truly uplifted and supported during one of the toughest moments of my life. It was a deeply vulnerable process for me to voice, but if there is one thing my life, my spirit, and my work in the world has taught me, it's that sharing helps it all feel less heavy. Just know that whatever "middle" you are currently navigating, you don't have to go through it alone, and you don't need to reach a pretty and perfect finish line to receive acknowledgment. We often praise people for their resilience instead of affirming that they did not deserve all they endured; that they are worthy of softness and rest and breaks from carrying it all. This is an important reframe in a world that always expects us to keep pushing through.

A GENTLE LOVE NOTE TO ALL THOSE WHO ARE EXHAUSTED BY RESILIENCE

Resilience doesn't always mean "powering through." It can also mean:

- Honoring the needs of the current season and remembering that it won't always be this hard
- Centering your mental health
- Celebrating your sensitivity
- Tending to yourself with extra care
- Nurturing relationships that help you feel seen and affirmed in your feelings
- Upholding your boundaries
- Doing nothing
- Receiving support
- Crying

A Meditation to Get Reacquainted with Your Needs and Vulnerabilities

Take as much time as you need to gently orient and set up your practice in any way that supports your ease, well-being, and care. You're welcome to complete this meditation in a chair or perhaps on a cushion on the floor. It might feel more supportive to rest on a couch or a bed. This is your practice and always your choice. Know that you can shift or make a change at any time to increase your comfort and allow for more ease, softness, and care.

To begin, I invite you to explore a mantra or an intention. Perhaps one like *I am enough; I allow myself to rest; I am wise, beautiful, and strong; I have so much goodness to give and receive*, or *I deserve to reclaim my care* might feel good to you. Take a moment to think about just how easy it is to go through an entire day being disconnected from your needs or unaware of all the ways your body is communicating with you. Usually when we're not in our bodies fully, we're in our minds. So I invite you to take a deep, full breath here, and on your exhale, allow yourself to relax a little bit deeper into your space to the degree that feels right and available to you.

Focus here on your mantra and the experience of feeling connected to your needs. Bring a level of awareness and mindfulness to those needs. Mindfulness allows us to pay attention with our whole mind and our whole hearts. It's a way for us to connect to the full resources of our body and our senses, taking note of what brings us joy, what brings us pleasure, and what allows us to feel supported.

So if it feels okay, I invite you to start to quiet your mind. Maybe become more aware of your breathing; perhaps exploring your neutral, compassionate breath at a pace that feels right and comfortable to you. If it's available, rest a palm on your heart and a palm on your belly, feeling the rise and fall of your beautiful, powerful breath. Feel free to observe any sensations that might be present for you. Know that all of you is welcome here.

Now explore what it would look like to honor your needs and vulnerabilities. Really start to shine light and bring awareness to how you would like to prioritize tending to yourself. Perhaps you'd like to schedule more restorative time into your days, or maybe you'd like to move yourself up to the top of your priority list. Continue to explore your inhales and exhales and allow yourself to rest and relax a little bit deeper, or even a little bit braver. Can you start to take note of where you might create a little more space for yourself in your day-to-day life? Can you carry that intention and energy with you as you navigate the ebbs and flows of your day?

In this space of intention and mindfulness, explore turning the volume of your heart all the way up and the volume of your thoughts all the way down. Allow the quiet and the stillness to reveal what you know to be true: You are worthy of your care. Your needs matter. You do not have to prioritize yourself last anymore. The intentional choices you make to choose yourself over and over again are necessary and important.

Take note of what it feels like in your body to take your time and not rush, to not respond to the urgency of others. What does it look like to turn down the needs of everyone else for a moment and spend time getting clarity around what you need? Take a deep, full inhale, then exhale with an open mouth. Take a few moments to settle back into your mantra now: *I am enough. I allow myself to rest. I am wise, beautiful, and strong. I have so much goodness to give and receive. I deserve to reclaim my care.* Feel free to find any final shape of rest that supports you. Take what you need here.

When you feel ready to move forward, bring some awareness back into your space and your body. Be gentle with your mind. Maybe you can start by wiggling your fingers or circling your wrists. You might explore wiggling your toes or circling your ankles and gently bringing your compassionate awareness back in. If you'd like, rest in a seated position with your palms together at the center of your heart, if that's a gesture that feels comfortable. Hands at your heart, may we live our lives compassionately. Hands at your mouth, may we speak words of truth and of kindness. And hands at your third-eye center, the light in me always honors the light in you. Namaste.

To access an audio recording of this meditation,
visit us.macmillan.com/ProtectYourEnergy.

. . . .

I hope this chapter has allowed you to see yourself in all of your humanness. Maybe there was a nugget of wisdom that resonated with your heart. I encourage you to write it down, savor the reminder, and continue to find your unique and gentle pace through it all. In the next chapter, we'll explore how embodied boundaries are foundational to everything we have explored together thus far.

4

Restoring the Nervous System Through Embodied Boundaries

You deserve to be in environments that bring out
the softness in you, not the survival in you.[1]
—RONNE BROWN

If you have ever attended a training or workshop with me or even
read my first book, *Trauma-Informed Yoga for Survivors: Practices for
Healing and Teaching with Compassion*, you may know that my favorite quote is attributed to Maya Angelou: "Your energy introduces
you before you even speak." These words have cascaded through
so many aspects of my life, and they often swirl around my brain
and body as an anchor. They are a constant reminder of why I am
passionate about centering and protecting my energy as an everyday
practice because of the palpable sense of "flow" the practice brings
into my life.

In positive psychology, flow is often referred to as "being in the
zone," a state one enters when they're so fully immersed and absorbed
in an enjoyable activity or task that they're able to be deeply present.
Every time I come back to Maya Angelou's words, I am reminded
of the ripple impact that our energy has on our well-being, our
parenting/caregiving, our relationships, our mental health, and
our ability to show up each and every day as our full selves. Embodied
boundaries are at the center of this truth because without them, we may
struggle to expend our energy with intention.

Boundaries can fall into many different categories: physical, emotional, professional, mental, sexual, capacity, time, and so many more as they relate to the ways we honor and uphold what feels most comfortable and aligned for us. For example, a physical boundary can be communicating your need for personal space or honoring your body's basic needs. An emotional boundary can be recognizing when you've reached your capacity for providing ongoing support for someone in your life and encouraging them with other resources, such as seeking mental health support. A professional boundary can be maintaining appropriate limits around your working hours, taking all of your designated time off and really honoring your out-of-office time, and answering emails during your working hours instead of constantly getting caught up in the urgency of others' requests.

Embodied boundaries allow us to integrate the head and the heart in this process. They are essentially how we attune to and honor our body's messages and responses, and how that informs our manner of communicating and asserting our needs. Embodied boundaries allow us to intentionally involve the mind, body, and spirit in our everyday experiences and interactions. This level of self-awareness is often cultivated through a practice of mindfulness and developing a strong and attuned relationship with our nervous system.

As we have learned, our bodies are always communicating to us (in subtle and not so subtle ways). We can learn to work with this sensory information and integrate it into our boundary-setting process. This is a sacred ecosystem. While the word *balanced* can feel charged to me (and I imagine many of us), we can lean in to the process of finding a gentle recalibration between our nervous system states without judgment, stigma, or shame. This is mirrored by the window-of-tolerance framework that we covered together in chapter 1. The goal isn't to put pressure on ourselves to be calm when our boundaries are challenged or pushed but rather to meet resistance and constriction with softness. This can help us prioritize the practices that help us anchor more wholly into our nuanced needs.

In her book *Choose You*, the therapist Helen Marie shares, "Noticing how I feel in relation to how much energy I have and who has access to my energy is an integral part of my ability to function optimally."[2]

How often do you mindfully check in with yourself and take stock of what energizes and drains you? Hopefully after what you've learned and practiced so far, it's more often than before. Marie says that energy drainers include "workload disagreements, poor sleep, too much screen time, comparison, perfectionism, other people's negativity, and lack of boundaries." Energy sources include "creativity, spending time with people who inspire and uplift you, long nourishing walks in nature, doing things that spark joy, or simply taking five minutes for yourself."[3] This chapter will focus on helping you further tune in to your body so you can make informed choices, set boundaries for what you invest your energy into, and prioritize the energy sources that benefit you most.

The Power of Embodied Boundaries

As participants arrived at one of my Healing in Community workshops, the first thing I shared was that showing up is so often the hardest part and that this was a space where they were not expected to hold it all together. It was a space where they could safely tend to their emotional armor and know that they were held. A space where the choices they made with their bodies were celebrated. A space where they didn't have to do any of the healing work alone (nor were they ever meant to). And a space where they could be abundantly gentle and honor the multiple truths of joy and grief that may be present at the same time.

As I gazed around the space, I could see the collective nervous systems in the room start to settle, as well as so many tears of release. The weight they all carried was palpable, but what was even stronger was the powerful energy shift that happened when they felt seen. Many of us have so few spaces where we can truly show up in all of our vulnerabilities, just as we are, so I wanted to ensure each and every participant felt supported from the moment we all came together.

An integral part of the embodied boundaries journey is attuning to the difference between having time versus having capacity. Just because we have time doesn't necessarily mean our nervous systems have the capacity to hold it all. When we are used to constantly pushing, we don't always honor our boundaries and allow ourselves the space to slow down and check in. You might look at your already very full day and think, *Sure, I can squeeze one more thing in*, when you are already on the brink of collapse. This is what the participants of my workshop had experienced, and finally having permission to relax and just be took a massive weight off their collective shoulders. My hope is that this chapter will have the same effect on you.

In her book *Permission to Rest*, the author Ashley Neese reminds us that "when our bodies are taxed from lack of rest, chronic stress, unaddressed trauma, discrimination, or hustle culture, we are more susceptible to illness."[4] We often treat rest as something we will do when we just have "more time." The challenge is this cumulative rest deficiency (and the constant borrowing of time from tomorrow) keeps us in stress-response cycles. My dear friend and colleague dr. shena young often describes energy depletion as feeling like someone literally plugged into you like you are an electrical outlet—a powerful visual that I imagine many of us can relate to in our own ways! This can make it even more difficult to have clarity around our boundaries and get honest with ourselves about where they are so deeply needed in our lives.

Dr. Nedra Glover Tawwab, the beloved boundary queen and *New York Times* bestselling author of *Set Boundaries, Find Peace*, shares in her chapter on the cost of not having healthy boundaries that "one of the biggest triggers for anxiety is the inability to say no."[5] This is why this chapter is dedicated to learning the *somatics* of boundaries and how integral it is to attune to the feedback our bodies give us. In her book, Dr. Tawwab shares the very real impact that a lack of boundaries can have on our mental health including neglecting self-care, worrying about what others think, overextending, not allowing others to help, and having high expectations of ourselves. This can lead to even further health impacts such as anxiety, depression, and physical symptoms of stress. She reminds folks to take stock of the following signs, as they may be an indication that more boundaries are needed:

- You feel overwhelmed.
- You feel resentful toward people for asking for your help.

- You avoid phone calls and interactions with people who might ask for something.
- You make comments about helping people and getting nothing in return.
- You feel burned out.
- You frequently daydream about dropping everything and disappearing.
- You have no time for yourself.[6]

Can you relate to any of these signs? If so, can you recall how they felt in your body? What words would you use to describe that very real, sensory experience (e.g., physically worn down, rage, difficulty sleeping, deep exhaustion, brain fog, headaches)? Can you think of a time when you had a conflict with someone and they said something that was so hurtful or made you so angry that your nervous system felt completely hijacked? Maybe you felt some combination of the fight, flight, or freeze response. When you experienced those moments, did you communicate that you were unable to continue the conversation? Did you give yourself space to decompress and regulate? Essentially, did you offer yourself the grace and compassion to take a time-out? As we unpacked in chapter 1, a big part of healing is reconnecting with your nervous system and being intentional about how you manage your stress. Can you see why leaving the body out of boundary work is incomplete? Abandoning yourself is no longer the way.

The Somatics of Boundaries

What I have found in my work as a trauma-informed educator is that approaching our boundaries from a nervous system–informed perspective can often be the missing link. Many of us fall into the trap of agreeing to things before we have adequately assessed our time and energy. As we discussed earlier, our tendency to do this is so intertwined with urgency culture; we think we need to respond to any and every request immediately or continue to stay in conversation with folks who are clearly making us uncomfortable instead of listening to our bodies. It took years of gastrointestinal issues for me to finally realize that my lack of boundaries not only increased my anxiety but also significantly impacted my physical health. The correlation seems so clear to me now, but in the thick of it, it was hard to make the connection.

Instead of acquiescing to requests or taking on more without taking stock of your capacity, I invite you to consider what your body is telling you and take note of how it lands and what might shift for you. If you need help coming up with questions to ask yourself in these moments, here are a few to get you started (feel free to add to this list):

- Does the thought of doing this deplete me or energize me?
- When I pause to take an embodied check-in of my current capacity, what comes up for me that may inform my decision?
- When I agree to this request, what other things am I also saying yes to that may be taxing for my mind, body, and spirit?
- Does this lift or add to the weight I am currently holding?
- If I do have time, do I also have the capacity?
- If I say yes to this, do I anticipate feeling resentful or having to potentially cancel later?
- If I take this on, what other areas of my life am I saying no to or neglecting?
- Does this need to happen now or can it wait until after I create more space for myself?
- How does taking this on support the health of my nervous system? Whenever possible, how can I be more discerning with my energy?
- Does the compensation I will receive accurately reflect the amount of work I'll do?
- What cues do I receive from my body when I envision taking this on? Sparkly and warm or constricted and uneasy?
- How might I be more intentional with what I commit to?
- What does it mean to honor my capacity and bandwidth as an ongoing, fluid, and changing practice?

There is a reason we repeatedly hear the phrase "trust your gut." In the simplest of terms, our bodies communicate through sensation. We often think about boundaries solely from a cognitive place, but boundaries—or a lack of them—can activate all parts of our being, and we need a more intentional and holistic approach in order to develop a sustainable set of practices for communicating them. When we can drop into our unique and tailored version of embodiment and nurture our boundaries from this place, they have the potential to open up space in our lives and allow us to access more freedom and self-care.

You may be surprised to learn that when your boundaries are crossed, you can feel it somatically in your body. These symptoms may include feeling physically ill when working in a toxic job/environment, getting a stomachache when thinking about having a conversation with someone who has been disrespectful, feeling jittery or anxious upon receiving a text from someone who does not value your time, or experiencing an emotional shutdown or freeze when your nervous system does not feel safe in a particular space.

Can you think of any other physiological impacts you experience when your boundaries are crossed or challenged? Or how about the various ways your body communicates that something is a "no" (e.g., a scratchiness in your throat, an uneasy feeling swirling around your stomach, body aches, shoulder tension, tightness in your chest, sweaty palms, a flushed face)? You deserve to pay attention to these sensations and no longer ignore them at the expense of your spirit and well-being.

Alternatively, how often do you pay attention to the ways your body communicates a "yes" (e.g., shoulders relax, an expansive and open feeling in your heart, butterflies of excitement, full-body joy, etc.)? What does your body experience in a space that feels safe for your nervous system? Perhaps this looks like a state of social engagement (pleasant smiles and compassionate eye contact), presence, connectedness, or ease. In my trauma-informed yoga certification trainings, we often talk about how body language is such a powerful indicator of comfort levels. This is a language all on its own that is worth our attention.

The Need for Boundaries

I have struggled with boundaries around my time, energy, capacity, relationships, and work my entire life, and there is no easy framework for unpacking the layers that I know are present for so many of us on this journey. I used to approach my boundaries solely from a cognitive place. (Why did I say yes to that project, and how did I end up this overwhelmed again?!) I inflicted a lot of shame upon myself for repeating patterns that left me exhausted and for not being able to get clear on my boundaries and stick to them. It should be easier than this, right?! I will tell you that berating myself was *not* the answer.

In many ways, I was disconnected from my spirit because of the weariness of life. My husband and I had been in a season that pushed us to our brink as we navigated fertility treatments and constant appointments, raising our six-year-old, staying on top of our businesses, trying to take care of ourselves and tend to each other's needs, feeling the heaviness of the world, working to stay connected to our support systems, and trying to function daily when life felt full. We nervously laughed with each other when we opened a fortune cookie one day and it said plain and simply, "Stop wearing yourself out." We felt seen and attacked at the same time!

Many of us may feel so run down from the perpetual chaos of being human that we sometimes lose sight of how to nurture and protect our own light. The shift for me happened when I started approaching and honoring my boundaries from an embodied lens. Accessing the depth of my sensory cues and paying attention to how they informed the way I honored myself and communicated what is in my heart has been a profound lesson to me that boundary work *is* nervous system work.

What I mean when I say this is that I couldn't cut myself off from the real physiological messages my body was sending me; I had to learn how to be in relationship with them. I don't think we talk enough about the physical sensations that can occur when we know we need to set a boundary and when we actually set them. If you are someone who has a highly sensitive nervous system, setting boundaries in this way can be particularly challenging and may require extra care, compassion, and space to decompress and process.

I know how difficult and overwhelming it can be to set boundaries and actually stick to them, especially if this is a new muscle you are building. You may feel pressured to continue overextending yourself so you don't disappoint others, but this is often at the expense of yourself and your mental health. I want to reassure you that it is okay if this process takes time for you. Just like there are no quick fixes to healing our nervous systems, the process of honoring your embodied boundaries will take an abundance of self-compassion, patience, and bravery. Over time and with repetition, the process will become easier for you. Additionally, the tools you accumulate throughout this book will continue to support you in exploring and getting more acquainted with your own needs so that honoring your embodied boundaries journey becomes more natural to you. When you recognize how necessary it is to honor and prioritize yourself, the ability to reclaim your own care becomes more manageable.

Boundary work is nervous system work.

Boundary work is nervous system work.

Boundary work is nervous system work.

Protecting our energy, taking care of ourselves, and setting boundaries are all interconnected. Setting boundaries becomes more manageable when our nervous systems are resourced because we have more capacity, grit (courage and resolve), and resilience to tend to the overwhelm that may surface in these moments. We have more space to reflect on our needs and how we'd like to communicate them. When I am overextended, overwhelmed, and consistently running myself ragged (and honestly in need of boundaries the most), it makes it harder to set them because I am so disconnected from myself. It makes it challenging to connect to that inner voice when everything else is so loud.

Have you ever noticed that when you communicate and assert your boundaries when you are burnt out or depleted, it can be challenging to articulate what wants to come through? Or maybe you say exactly what you want to say but not always with the grace you might have hoped for. This is because our nervous systems may be stuck in a sympathetic, or stressed, state. When we set boundaries in that expanded window-of-tolerance space, it can allow us to communicate from the most authentic version of ourselves.

You are allowed to take time to pour into yourself, love. Choosing not to rush yourself is a beautiful way of honoring your boundaries. And you know what? Sometimes giving yourself grace looks like letting the anger come through just as it is. There is no one-size-fits-all approach, just layers upon layers of honoring our unique lived experiences.

When I am well resourced, I can communicate with more grace.

Reconnecting to Your Nervous System

Building my nervous system capacity has also increased my ability to tend to the discomfort that arises when I need to set boundaries and offer myself more gentleness. My body is the first to alert me when I'm out of my window of tolerance—usually in the form of agitation! This intimate relationship with my nervous system capacity is a constantly evolving process, but things that help me cultivate a more supportive and nourishing relationship with myself include:

- Being intentional about screen time limits and putting my phone on Do Not Disturb
- Monitoring how much of myself I give away during the day
- Letting ten minutes of yoga be enough
- Waking up before my family for some quiet alone time
- Listening to something uplifting or restorative, instead of the news, on my way to work
- Honoring my body and letting myself rest when I need to
- Romanticizing the small joys of my life
- Treating my morning coffee as a spiritual practice and sacred ritual

- Doing work that fulfills me and feeds my soul
- Taking my joy seriously
- Practicing community care
- Saying no more often
- Paying attention to when my nervous system communicates a yes or no
- Practicing intentional emotional regulation
- Hiking and spending time in nature
- Letting myself get lost in the present moment with my children
- Unplugging from my phone
- Getting to the root of any resentment
- Being consistent with therapy

So much of the process of reconnecting to my nervous system is about increasing my bandwidth and building resilience in small ways throughout the day. It's committing to rituals (while also being flexible) and being intentional about my choices in order to minimize my habit of consistently living in a state of hyperarousal. I'm human, so I don't always get it right or do these things consistently. But having these core values, practices, and anchors to help me recalibrate sets the foundation for me to uphold and honor my boundaries more than I used to.

Building my nervous system capacity in this way has also increased my ability to tend to the uneasiness that would arise from being perceived as "rude" when really I was just honoring what was within my current capacity (a gift not only to myself but to others in my life). You can be a kind person and still set clear boundaries. These two things are not mutually exclusive. Setting boundaries is a self-love practice that ripples and radiates. When we are grounded in our boundaries and truth, we mirror and model the practice for others, which makes it more accessible, attainable, and normalized. It becomes an integrated part of our relationships that facilitates trust. Imagine if we were able to consistently model this type of self-care to our loved ones, including our children. The results would likely be collectively transformative.

As we explored earlier, the overstimulation, overscheduling, and overriding of our nervous system cues and boundaries starts from a young age. Children are constantly navigating various fight, flight, and freeze states in the school systems that train them to rush and achieve more; rarely are they modeled the gifts of stillness and spaciousness. Their schedules are often packed with activities, nonstop assignments, and rushed meals. In the end, we work so hard in adulthood to untangle from these messages. For those who have never had healthy boundaries modeled to them through words or actions or who have repeatedly had their boundaries violated by people who were supposed to care for them, it is completely understandable why you may struggle with honoring your needs.

In her book *Good Inside*, the clinical psychologist Dr. Becky Kennedy talks about the concept of "unformulated experience," which is the feeling many of us get that something is off or not right without an honest or clear explanation of why. She shares how terrifying this can be for children because that feeling "free-floats around the body without an anchor of safety." She reminds us that "when kids are left to make sense of a scary change on their own, they usually rely on the methods that give them control: self-blame ('I must have done something to cause this. I'm bad, I'm too much') and self-doubt ('I must have misunderstood the tension around me. I am not such a good feeler of things. If something really was different, my parents would explain it to me')."[7] So much of this tension around trusting ourselves can be carried with us into adulthood. This is one of the many reasons honoring the needs of our inner child and our many versions can be so healing.

Part of generational and community healing is being able to carve out a new path of liberation for ourselves. And because there are so many systemic factors out of our control, being intentional with normalizing boundaries and modeling them for others to build consistent anchors of safety is a great path forward. It's a way to reclaim so many parts of ourselves that have been swept up in emotional labor and the persistent and ongoing demands of it all.

Nurturing Your Embodied Boundaries

Boundaries are the distance at which I can
love you and me simultaneously.[8]
—PRENTIS HEMPHILL

The following practice can be helpful in the moments when you feel in your body that you need to set a boundary or when you're going through the often challenging and conflicting process of actually setting one. As always, be gentle with yourself and any emotions that might surface during your practice.

To begin, I invite you to take a deep, full inhale and a long, slow exhale—your pace, your way. No need to control or constrict the breath in any way. Honor it just as it is. Throughout this practice, I encourage you to keep this mantra in mind: *My boundaries guide me to wholeness and truth. I give up freely what no longer serves me. I release it to create space for what inspires me.*

Gently find your way into any shape that allows you to feel supported and nourished. You're welcome to find a seat in a chair, on the couch, or even on your bed. You might place a cushion on the floor and find a seated meditation. Or you could lie down on your back or gently rest on your belly, allowing your face to fall to one side. If there is any other shape of relaxation that feels better today, please honor that. If you'd like, you could also bring some awareness to your heart space, perhaps resting your palms there for a moment, if it feels okay and available to you.

In this space of ease, I invite you to explore breathing into your spirit and your beautiful light. Can you allow your breath to rest a little deeper? Tune inward and find gentle compassion and love for your practice today. Perhaps take note of the beautiful sound of your breath. How can your mantra be a guide to help you cultivate the strength and clarity you need to set important boundaries in your life? Feel free to come back to it when you feel called to: *My boundaries guide me to wholeness and truth. I give up freely what is no longer serving me. I create space for what inspires me.*

If it feels okay, rub your palms together, creating some warmth, and then gently rest them over the heart or on any parts of the body that need your attention, mindfulness, support, intention, and care. Can you feel the warmth radiating within? Allow it to be a reminder of the beauty of your boundaries; the beauty of being intentional with your energy, time, and care.

If you'd like, I invite you to extend that energy and intention high to the sky, perhaps extending your fingertips up, moving your intention there and holding it for a moment. Take note of a sense of grounding beneath you, a sense of feeling held and supported, and let that be a reminder that you are never alone in your experience. Take note of the energy of feeling rooted, of feeling grounded, as you simultaneously lift your intention and connect to your inner sense of strength. To your boundaries, your care, your energy.

Holding your intention here, allow yourself to be in the light. Notice the energy sparkling from your fingertips. Take a moment to anchor yourself back into the mantra: *My boundaries guide me to wholeness and truth. I give up freely what is no longer serving me. I create space for what inspires me.* Linger here for as long as you need.

Whenever you feel ready, I invite you to reach your fingertips toward the sky once again on your next inhale, then exhale and push your palms out and away from your body. This is a symbolic gesture of releasing energy that does not serve you, a moment to honor your sense of embodied boundaries. Repeat this as many times as it feels supportive to you.

On your next exhale, gently release your palms and rest them anywhere on your body that feels supportive. Relax your shoulders back and down your spine and take note of the sound of your breath. Notice what it feels like in your body to make intentional choices around your boundaries, time, and energy. Pause here to honor all that you hold, all that you do, all that you navigate daily. Ground yourself here in your worthiness. Feel that embodied sense of strength that you cultivate within your body. Relax deeply into this space, and let anything that does not serve you roll off of your shoulders. Let this be a reminder that you are never alone in what you are navigating.

Before we close out this practice, I invite you to consider what boundaries are calling out to you and revealing themselves. How can you embody a new way of approaching your day that honors your time and energy? If it feels okay, I invite you to envision a beautiful shining light circling around you, your space, and your practice. Can you visualize this as a protective boundary, fiercely protecting and honoring your light, energy, and personal boundaries? Know you're worthy of staying in the light, of honoring the preciousness of your being and your care. Know that there are many pathways to healing, and your boundaries deserve to be prioritized.

As we slowly bring this practice to a close, you are welcome to keep your eyes open, find a soft gaze, or close them. Spend some time in quiet reflection and journal about what came up for you, of maybe one tangible boundary that you'd like to set or ideas for protecting your energy. Know that everything you are feeling is so valid and absolutely welcome in this space. These moments of resistance deserve to be met with compassion and care as opposed to just being pushed through. I'll leave you here in this moment of quiet reflection. Take all the time you need.

To access an audio recording of this meditation,
visit us.macmillan.com/ProtectYourEnergy.

As we close out this chapter, I want to leave you with a few reminders on your boundaries journey. First, every time you honor your boundaries, you are protecting your mental health. In a world that constantly demands more from us, being intentional and discerning with our energy is our most powerful resource. Next, your unmet needs are often a source of energy depletion, which can lead to irritability, stress, and burnout. You are worthy of centering your needs and setting boundaries that protect and even heal your nervous system. And finally, nervous system health is a foundational practice to being human in these times. You have full permission to honor your humanity and handle yourself with grace and care.

In the next chapter, I will build upon this lesson on the somatics of boundaries by offering a holistic road map to help you unwind from burnout. We've tackled some challenging topics thus far, and it's likely that uncomfortable emotions or sensations have come up during your meditation practices. If you are noticing your body is in need of a break or simply space to decompress, please flip to the practices in chapters 6 or 7 at any time. You don't need to move through the content in a linear fashion. Take what you need, love.

5

A Mind, Body, and Spirit Approach to Unwinding from Burnout

I know you squeeze into tight spaces with the hope that you may fit without aching. There are spaces meant for you that will not require you to bend in order to belong safely.[1]
—BRIANNA PASTOR

Dr. Ann Masten, a researcher who specializes in resilience and development, refers to the phenomenon of our system working in overdrive as "surge capacity depletion," sharing that this is a "collection of adaptive systems—mental and physical—that humans draw on for short-term survival in acutely stressful situations."[2] In other words, we tend to cling to whatever we can to simply get through. This is one of the reasons why burnout accumulates in sometimes sneaky and unexpected ways, often over long periods of time, and the residual impacts and memories tend to live in the body.

In their book *Burnout: The Secret to Unlocking the Stress Cycle*, burnout experts Emily and Amelia Nagoski share, "We get stuck in the stress response because we're stuck in a stress-activating situation. That's not always bad—it's only bad when the stress outpaces our capacity to process it."[3] They explain that our stress response cycle is "a biological process in our bodies that has a beginning, middle, and end." Examples of things that might activate our stress response cycle on a daily basis include traffic and long commutes, caregiving with no support, unsustainable or overwhelming workloads, an inability to tend to our personal needs, systemic oppression, and relentless news cycles, to name a few. The goal, of course, is to recognize when your stress response is triggered, then remedy it with soothing practices that can bring you back to your center.

The practices offered in this book can support you in completing the stress cycle you might be navigating in your life so that you can avoid burnout and keep your nervous system in a parasympathetic, or ventral vagal, state. Luckily, completing your stress cycle doesn't have to be complicated. Small things such as movement, a twenty-second hug from a safe and trusted person, and sleep can all work wonders in reducing stress levels and bringing you back to a calm baseline.[4]

Getting more attuned to our stress response system is powerful because our stress plays such a pivotal role in keeping us safe, but it's important to remember that we are not meant to live in survival mode for long periods of time. In their book *The Secret Language of the Body*, the mind and body practitioners Jennifer Mann and Karden Rabin share that when stress builds up, it can lead to what scientists refer to as the allostatic load, "a term referring to the cumulative effects of chronic stress and life events on the body. A high allostatic load strains your body's ability to regulate itself and return to a state of balance. At the cellular level, this strain brings about changes that impact energy production, immune function, hormone signaling and cellular repair, ultimately affecting overall health."[5]

Making yourself a priority and finding ways to actively process your stress can positively impact every aspect of your life; the ripple effects are endless. Additionally, the buffers of rest (more on this in the next chapter) that you start to integrate throughout your day can help you cultivate positive stress responses, allowing you to better handle the daily stressors of life and avoid the negative effects of burnout. Most importantly, what works to support the regulation of your nervous system may be different from what works for someone else. There is no one-size-fits-all approach. As Abby Rawlinson shared on Instagram, "Regulation doesn't always look like slowing down.

Sometimes it looks like play. Or movement. Or laughing so hard you cry. Follow what brings aliveness—not just stillness."

In this chapter we'll spend time getting to the root of our burnout, understanding our habitual patterns, finding new ways to soften the intensity, and most importantly viewing all of this through a whole-body lens in order to make more informed choices around our energy.

Addressing Inner Resentment, Emotional Imprints, and Moving Beyond Survival

Overextending our energy is not the only thing that can result in burnout. In fact, leading from a place of resentment as opposed to fullness can be one of the quickest roads to burnout, which is, on a deeper level, a form of systems betrayal. The psychiatrist Pooja Lakshmin explores the concept of societal and systems betrayal in her book *Real Self-Care*, reminding us that while burnout places the blame and responsibility on the individual, betrayal points to the broken structures around them. She validates that bearing the mental load of all of this has serious emotional and psychological consequences.[6] In our most trying moments, we might be holding it together on the outside but crumbling on the inside. If this struggle feels familiar, please know you are not alone.

If you are just beginning the journey of unwinding from burnout, remind yourself with the utmost compassion that adopting a slower pace takes time. Amanda Perera shares, "Recovery from mental, emotional, or physical burnout can take years. Even if you start prioritizing rest and start living a softer life, your nervous system remembers the burnout and/or the trauma. Understanding this and being gentle and patient with ourselves is key."[7] In a world that wants to offer a quick solution to every life challenge, the work we're doing here together is from the inside out and from the root, which is truly the most sustainable and loving solution. It's about taking an honest look at the most tender parts of ourselves and acknowledging what needs have been neglected, what parts of the body need attention and support, and what it actually looks like to take up and reclaim space in what may feel like the mundane moments of life. The truth is those are the sacred moments that offer an opening to the lightness and ease you have been seeking. You deserve to truly live and not just survive, love.

As you begin to explore your relationship with burnout in this chapter and cultivate a more intentional relationship with your energy, I invite you to take note of what energies and responsibilities you might be carrying that are not yours. There are two powerful inquiries I shared in my first book that continue to offer me a soft place to land: "Are you carrying or caring?"[8] and "Are you absorbing or observing?"[9] How do these land for you? Take note of anything that might be coming up to the surface, and know that everything you feel is valid and welcome in this space.

Folks who tend to carry and absorb the energies of others are, according to the psychologist Bo Forbes, experiencing empathy as a form of emotional and sensory contagion.[10] This is a major source of energy depletion and can quickly lead to burnout and other health impacts. It turns out the more empathetic we are, the more likely we are to absorb other people's feelings and emotions as if they were our own. In yogic philosophy, emotional imprints like these that live in the body are called vasanas.[11] When vasanas remain undigested, they can get deep-rooted, hardwired, or lodged in various parts of the body, depending on the nature of what we have experienced, and can lead to stress responses, physical illness, and other somatic-based symptoms.

An example of this is if you grew up feeling like you always had to achieve or strive for perfection. When your "enoughness" feels challenged later in life, this can show up as symptoms such as stomachaches, an urge to overwork, or even panic attacks. The undigested sensory residue that accumulates in our bodies over time—whether it be stress, grief, trauma, or unmet needs—wants to be processed. Sometimes it may bubble up to the surface as rage, sadness, overwhelm, or physical symptoms, and all of these are valid. Regardless of how it presents, your body is communicating with you, urging you to notice the parts that need tending.

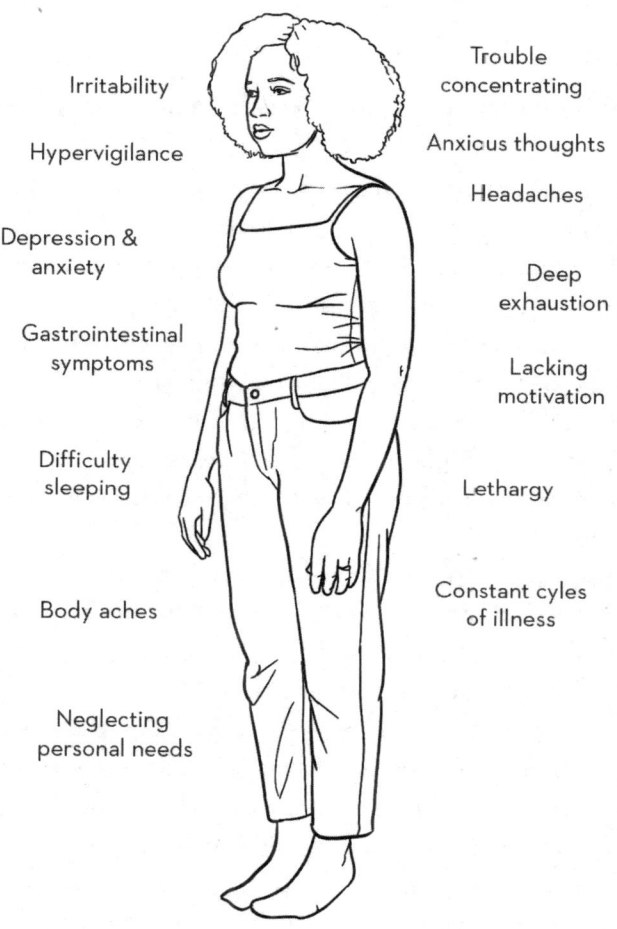

Irritability

Hypervigilance

Depression & anxiety

Gastrointestinal symptoms

Difficulty sleeping

Body aches

Neglecting personal needs

Trouble concentrating

Anxious thoughts

Headaches

Deep exhaustion

Lacking motivation

Lethargy

Constant cyles of illness

Burnout can manifest somatically in a variety of ways.

Luckily for us, when we slow down enough to listen to our body's wisdom, it can reveal so much. This is why engaging in body-based practices and adopting a slower pace (which we'll explore in the next few chapters) is so important. It allows us to gently tend to our vasanas and bring them to the surface so that we can begin the process of completing our stress cycle and befriending our nervous system.

Healing from Burnout and Toxic Work Environments

This meditation practice focuses on helping you heal from burnout and toxic work environments. Because we spend so much of our time at work, I've found that addressing this source of stress head-on can offer significant relief that echoes into the other aspects of our lives. A mantra that I have come back to almost every single day over the course of the past few years is from Dr. Susana Muñoz, an associate professor and researcher specializing in the experiences of minoritized populations in higher education: *I am not behind or unproductive. I'm doing as much as my mind and body are allowing me to do under perpetual stress and fatigue.*[12]

To begin, I invite you to take a deep, full inhale in and an exhale out at your pace and in your way. Explore your breath in a way that feels supportive and spacious to you, and know that you can come back to this breath and mantra at any time.

This practice is about offering yourself the compassion and grace you deserve amid all the trying moments you have been navigating. Be gentle with yourself as you start to slowly reacquaint with your breath. Can you melt a little bit deeper into your space? As you settle in—whether that's on a mat, a cushion, your bed, or the couch—know that your choices are absolutely celebrated here and you are free to make any shifts or changes that feel supportive.

If at any time throughout your practice you are met with overwhelming internal thoughts or sensations, you are welcome to explore the exteroceptive sensations in the space around you, something outside of your body. Maybe that is looking out the window at nature, taking note of something in your space that brings you a sense of ease or joy, or taking in your own compassion. Anything that would support you in safely reorienting back to your body is perfect.

Now, when you're comfortable and settled, I invite you to rest a palm on your heart and a palm on your belly and notice the rise and fall of your beautiful, powerful breath. Take a moment here to connect to an anchor, an inner resource, a supportive mantra, or an intention for your practice. What do you need a little bit more of in this moment? What brought you to this particular practice today? Can you take note of what is holding and supporting you here? Know that you are never alone in your struggle. Deeply feel and believe that you are held in community with those who see your struggle, who honor your lived experience, and who wish you peace and deep rest.

Remind yourself often that you are healing, even when it's hard. That every intentional choice you make to choose you matters. That reclaiming your care is an act of resistance. That burnout is not a badge of honor, that you deserve peace, that you deserve for others to acknowledge how hard it's been.

In this space of grace and acceptance, explore softening your breath, relaxing your shoulders down your spine, and letting any tension dissolve. Take a deep, full inhale and an open-mouth exhale. Can you slow your pace and be present with each inhale and each exhale?

As you continue to rest with your breath, I want to share a few reminders for you when resting feels hard. Feel free to rest your palms on any parts of the body that feel supportive to allow these words to land.

- You don't have to earn your rest.
- You are worthy and enough, just as you are.
- Your productivity does not determine your worth.
- You are worthy when you are at capacity.
- You are worthy when you need support.
- You are worthy when you're struggling.
- You are worthy of taking your time.
- You are worthy of your care.
- You are worthy when you don't have the bandwidth to support others.
- You are worthy of being seen.
- You are worthy of taking up space.
- You are worthy of appreciation.
- You are worthy when you break down.
- You are worthy when you're overwhelmed.
- You are worthy of ease and space.

- You are worthy of tending to your mental health.
- You are worthy of grace, compassion, support, affirmation, and understanding.
- You are worthy of joy, and it is safe to let it in.
- You are worthy of fun.
- You are worthy of love.
- You are worthy when you're resting.
- You are worthy when you choose you.

In this moment, I invite you to breathe all of that in. And, with an open-mouth exhale, release any lingering tension. Rest here for as long as you'd like in this space of worthiness and acceptance.

Now start to bring a little bit of movement into your body and space. You could gently circle your wrists or wiggle your fingers if that's accessible to you. You could bring some movement to your toes or circle your ankles. On your inhale, gently extend your arms high to the sky. If it feels okay, interlace your fingers and find the length through your spine all the way up through the crown of your head. Explore a gentle stretch side to side. Just notice that length and engagement on the sides of your body, only bending and stretching as deeply as feels accessible to you today.

In your time and in your way, place both of your palms on the top of your head and take another round of breath. Inhale and exhale. Inhale to invite your left palm over your forehead, and exhale to bring your right palm over your heart. Inhale, place your left palm over your belly, and exhale, place your right palm over your left. Take a moment here to reconnect to your intention, your mantra, your anchor: *I am not behind or unproductive. I'm doing as much as my mind and body are allowing me to do under perpetual stress and fatigue.* Continue these compassion holds for as long as feels good for you.

As we reach the end of this practice, you're welcome to rest your palms anywhere on your body or release them beside you. Take a moment here to check back in with yourself and ground into your worthiness. Continue breathing, finding more space and expansion.

When you feel ready, gently bring your palms together at the center of your heart or find any other expression or gesture that feels available and accessible to you. Hands at your heart, may we live our lives compassionately. Hands at your mouth, may we speak words of truth and kindness. And hands at your third-eye center, the light in me always honors the light in you. Namaste.

This meditation offered a lot of points of reflection, so I encourage you to be gentle with yourself and take some time to journal, process, and integrate whatever came up. Sending you so much love, care, and compassion. You are not alone in your experience.

To access an audio recording of this meditation,
visit us.macmillan.com/ProtectYourEnergy.

Ease Is a Daily Practice

Dorcas Cheng-Tozun, the author of *Social Justice for the Sensitive Soul*, describes a personal experience that I imagine many of us have our own tender version of:

> Like an ice shelf that suddenly collapses into the sea after years of unseen melting and fracturing, my breakdown had actually been a long time coming. I had spent years trying to be an idealized version of myself—working long hours, pushing myself in challenging roles, never saying no, and regularly placing myself in the contexts that petrified me. When my body communicated stress, I ignored it; I didn't listen to my heart when it ached from pain, sorrow, and exhaustion.[13]

I imagine we all can relate to that moment when the unraveling begins to take shape from years of suppressing our feelings, pushing through exhaustion and burnout, or ignoring our bodies' warning signs. As I'm sure many of you know, when we ignore these signals for too long, our bodies will eventually force us to take a break because they have run out of options. Prolonged states of hypervigilance and the corresponding stress take a significant toll on the body, and you deserve so much peace. Can you think of a time in your life when you realized your energy was completely depleted and you could no longer continue on? Be gentle with yourself as you recall the details of this time. All of this embodied wisdom supports your process of protecting your energy.

I remember the first time several years ago when my husband told me, with so much love and kindness, that he felt like I rarely had any "good energy" left for him at the end of the day. It was so crushing to hear him say this, but it was also a wake-up call. Even though I knew a lot of my overwhelm was due to the larger systems that enfold us, I knew there was more I could be doing to protect my energy, renew my approach to work, ask for help, and assert my boundaries so I could have enough overflow for my family *and* myself. I didn't want to get stuck in a shame cycle, and I certainly didn't enjoy the irritable and short-fused version of myself I came home with because I had given *all* of myself away at work. That reminder alone began to shift so many things for me.

So I want to say it again and speak directly to you: *You do not have to give all of yourself away during the day.* By portioning our energy like we practiced earlier, we can really start to embody ease as a daily practice. It is an act of community care to not normalize exhaustion. We all deserve so much more than the way we may be navigating our days in consistent cycles and patterns of depletion. We deserve to be more intentional with how we are using our energy, giving ourselves more space to soften and just be. It's important to ground ourselves in the fact that when we take the steps to heal and repair our relationship with our nervous systems, the positive impacts ripple out to all those we love and cherish.

I have had to forgive myself over and over for all of the times I tried to heal my burnout with quick fixes instead of sustainable practices, values, and boundaries. It turns out embodying a more restful way of being honors and centers our needs and requires support, compassion, tenderness, care, time, and patience—the same way physical and emotional healing does. When we find rest difficult or when overworking has become a relied-upon coping strategy, we often take on additional self-blame and pressure as a side effect. But we are worthy of treating rest like resistance and acknowledging the systems of oppression that have made rest inaccessible for so long. The systems we currently live under were never set up for us to thrive, which is why reclaiming our care is the strongest path to liberating our minds, bodies, and spirits.

In a world that makes it challenging to switch off the constant activation of the sympathetic nervous system, saying no, releasing urgency, choosing yourself, prioritizing your needs, and honoring your right to rest are courageous acts of resilience. In quiet moments of reflection, I often get sad when I think about all the time I lost living in survival mode. Then I remember how beautiful, expansive, and tangible healing can be. It opens up possibilities and pathways that once felt impossible. May we all ground ourselves in this truth as we navigate these nonlinear routes.

The Physiology of Burnout

In her book *Heal Your Nervous System*, Dr. Linnea Passaler, a medical professional and researcher, shares an incredibly helpful diagram for understanding the impact burnout can have on a sensitive nervous system. She shares that people with a sensitive nervous system are often prone to the burnout cycle because when their energy feels solid and balanced, they end up "taking on all of the things." Because their energy feels good, they don't keep track of how much they are taking on and they tend to overcommit, leading to a cycle that generally looks like this:

- Phase 1: Feels energized and overcommits
- Phase 2: Starts feeling overwhelmed
- Phase 3: Withdraws and shuts down
- Phase 4: Starts feeling better[14]

I don't know about you, but the first time I discovered this framework, I felt so seen. I spent years living in this cycle before I became

THE BURNOUT CYCLE
in the Sensitive Nervous System

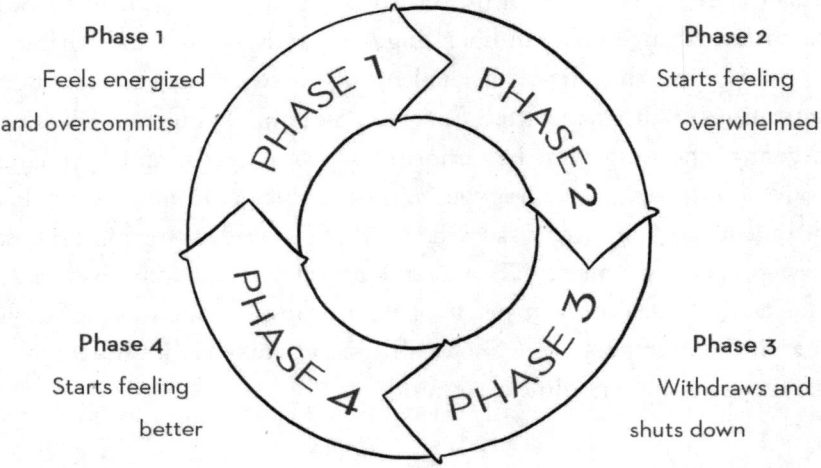

Phase 1

Feels energized and overcommits

Phase 2

Starts feeling overwhelmed

Phase 4

Starts feeling better

Phase 3

Withdraws and shuts down

Burnout occurs in a cycle for everyone but can affect those with highly sensitive nervous systems in specific ways.

more attuned to my nervous system and portioning my energy versus my time.

After becoming aware of this burnout cycle, I began to take my healing journey seriously and committed to the hard inner work of recognizing where I had been ignoring my body's warning signs. There are a few things that have stayed with me from my healing journey that I'd like to share with you.

- It is possible to create an intentional life that allows you to do work that you love without abandoning yourself. We have so many beautiful dimensions to us that deserve to be explored and tended to. Your needs matter, and they do not need to be sacrificed. The shift into this mindset starts with you believing in and honoring the parts of you that are craving to be seen.

- My therapist reminded me that the job I had may have provided stability in some ways, but the stability of my mental health deserved to be given the same amount of space and consideration in my mind. This gave me the courage to shift my focus to the next opportunity instead of staying in a toxic place, holding on to the false hope that things would get better if I just continued on as usual.
- Choosing to unapologetically tend to and honor your mental health may be incredibly uncomfortable, but you deserve to do it anyway.
- When you begin making intentional choices to honor your worth and value, people will not always be on board, and some of your relationships may change. This can incite its own type of grief. Be gentle with yourself. It's okay to prioritize your needs and stay firm in your boundaries.
- Burnout is real, and it is *not* your fault. Keep trusting in yourself, follow the signs your body is giving you, and know that peace awaits you. You are worthy of your healing. You're not alone.
- You won't always get the external validation and appreciation you may hope for. You deserve to be in spaces where you do not have to constantly hustle to prove your worth. Peace is possible. You are enough.
- Gaslighting, as well as the detrimental impact it can have on your spirit, is real. It is not just in your head. You deserve so much better.
- You can love what you do and also know that you are more than your work.
- You deserve a sustained presence of peace in your life.

I encourage you to keep these insights in mind as you navigate your healing journey from burnout. It can certainly sneak up on you without you being aware, but this is why tuning in to your body's cues and listening to what it tells you is so vitally important in your long-term energetic healing and your ability to set strong boundaries.

As we prepare to switch gears to the embodied practices and tools you can take with you on your healing journey, I invite you to refer to the following chart. It consolidates a lot of the concepts covered in the book so far and serves as a loving reminder of the various ways you can approach your healing through a mind, body, and spirit lens.

MIND	BODY	SPIRIT
Not blaming self when systems are at fault	Committing to a manageable workload	Practicing embodied boundaries
Practicing self-compassion	Giving your best vs. all; not giving all of yourself away during the day	Practicing energy protection
Lowering expectations for yourself and others	Prioritizing rest	Honoring your capacity as a core practice
Taking breaks from the mental load; asking for tangible support	Cultivating a slower pace and doing less	Gaining clarity around your values

In the next chapter, we will synthesize everything we've learned so far and focus on the various types of rest our nervous system needs. You will be invited to think outside the box when it comes to how you typically view rest. Keep an open mind and an open heart. I can't wait to explore this together.

6

The Intentional Practice of Rest

Maybe we don't need to be working harder,
but softer and more intentional.[1]
—MANASSALINE COLEMAN

My arms grew tired of constantly
reaching so I wrapped them around
myself and allowed them to rest.[2]
—L. E. BOWMAN

During an online training session, Tracee Stanley, the author of *Radiant Rest*, shared something quite interesting that happens often at her yoga retreats. When she invites folks to set up a Yoga Nidra practice for someone else, they tend to grab extra pillows, blankets, bolsters, socks, eye masks, and other props to provide maximum support, nourishment, and comfort. However, when she invites them to set up a yoga practice for themselves, they typically skip the props and offer themselves the bare minimum of support.[3] What a powerful metaphor for the care we so freely and enthusiastically pour into others but not always into ourselves.

This chapter is about leaning in to and offering yourself permission to receive the care, compassion, rest, and comfort you have been yearning for and deserve. You'll have an opportunity to reflect on the different types of rest your body needs, and I'll introduce you to some trauma-informed yoga shapes you can explore when you feel exhausted. As a gentle reminder before we begin: It's okay to honor the way your body is communicating with you about its need for deep rest. You don't need to intellectualize it or figure out why you feel the way you do. Trust that your body knows exactly what it needs and do your best to honor its requests. You are so worthy.

Rest Is Always Available

We live in a world that constantly affirms that our worth as humans is directly tied to our productivity. As a result, there is limited language around how integral restoration, ease, and embodied boundaries are to functioning in such a demanding way. As we've learned, practicing self-consent or an embodied check-in before you overextend your energy is one way (of many) to avoid overriding the messages of your nervous system and I encourage you to embrace this as a daily sacred practice.

But I, of course, honor and recognize that many of us work in professions that don't offer a lot of flexibility due to set and standard appointments, schedules, and responsibilities. Others of us may be navigating the near-constant demands of caregiving on top of the myriad worries, anxieties, stressors, and challenges we hold as we move through our days. Some may be moving through health challenges that feel invisible, dismissed, or heavy to carry.

Class intersects every aspect of these choices because when you are living paycheck to paycheck or are faced with unrelenting responsibilities, resting and making intentional choices around your schedule may feel completely unattainable. The researcher and author Ximena Vengoechea shares that we need "systemic solutions to prevent the exhaustion and fatigue so many of us feel today, like having universal healthcare, universal daycare, paid family leave, better sick leave policies, stronger rights for disabled people, experimental community housing design, and a universal basic income."[4] While we can't always quickly create the systemic change we desperately need and deserve, we *can* certainly impact the system from the inside out.

The ways we care for ourselves are revolutionary in a system that thrives on our exhaustion. Embodying this is, in fact, what shifts culture.

It creates a pathway for adults and children alike to know all the options of care, softness, and rest that are available to them. It affirms that working ourselves into the depths of exhaustion is not the only way. In doing so, we both honor the role of rest in our lives and can model it for others (children, partners, parents, coworkers, and friends). This, in and of itself, can be a deeply healing and transformative process as it works to shift cultural and generational patterns.

When I FaceTime my parents only to find them napping in the middle of the day, I can't help but have the biggest smile on my face. This is something I rarely witnessed growing up. My parents immigrated to the US from India with eight dollars in their pockets after my dad finished pharmacy school. In doing so, they experienced challenges in acclimating and finding their way to becoming business owners in California. My dad worked Monday through Saturday and my mom was an accountant who did all of the bookkeeping for him. She still managed to never miss my and my sister's games, shuttle us around to all of our activities, be present for homework and meltdowns, make the most delicious Indian meals, and insert magic into just about everything in our lives. So much of my work ethic and parenting philosophy comes from them and how they modeled that anything is possible when you believe in yourself.

My dad's entrepreneurial spirit will always live in my bones, and I can't help but smile when he asks me "what exactly" I do during a sabbatical (something I never thought could be a reality for me due to grind culture). I find these moments with him so sweet and endearing, and it allows us to have generative conversations that show that cycles can change. That healing and rest are possible. That our productivity does not determine our worth. That our bodies are worth the pause to simply be in whatever way we have the capacity to make space for.

In my adult life, it has taken several years and lessons for me to venture out of the traditional norms of productivity to support my mental health. I have an overachieving work ethic (I think this will always be hard to untangle from), but I simultaneously opt for more restoration and rest wherever I can grasp it. I remember one of my best friends telling me how solid my boundaries are and how much she appreciates that in both my work and personal lives I practice what I preach. It was one of the sweetest compliments, and it allowed me to acknowledge how much time and healing this type of growth has taken me.

In daily practice, this type of growth can be demonstrated in the way we embody a slower pace, how intentional we are with what we commit to, how we limit overscheduling or overstimulating ourselves, and how we prioritize creating space in our day. **Being constantly busy and stressed is not the marker of success we've been told it is.**

Tricia Hersey's work speaks to this almost exclusively and is deeply meaningful and impactful. In her *New York Times* bestselling book *Rest Is Resistance*, she shares how "grind culture has normalized pushing our bodies to the brink of exhaustion" and that "sleep deprivation is a racial and social justice issue." She reminds us that "resting is a connection and a path back to our true nature" and powerfully declares that "our bodies don't belong to these toxic systems . . . and our Spirits know better."[5] Her persevering voice in this movement encourages us to be curious about the type of deep rest and care our souls need and to resist the societal messaging that pressures us to grind at the expense of our bodies.

The message here is that rest is always available to us, especially in the small pockets of time where we can resist the urge to be in constant states of output. But as I mentioned, committing to rest, even in small ways, is not always an easy choice. Instead, this work requires a deep internal commitment to yourself and the recognition that your rest trickles out into the collective. Shifting our culture's view of rest is about recognizing the humanity in each of us, choosing ourselves, tenderly caring for our well-being, and shifting blame for our burnout to the systems that create the unjust conditions and barriers to rest.

In her book *All the Gold Stars*, the freelance writer and reporter Rainesford Stauffer talks about the ways we can reimagine ambition and shares her own trying moment: "I handed over pieces of me to sketchy bosses who had me working 39.5 hours to avoid granting health insurance, which turned out to be a dire trade-off . . . as my physical and mental health demanded my attention, I attempted to work around them, to patch holes in myself."[6] Reading her experience made me recall all the times I was praised in the workplace for overachieving while I was also extremely depressed, anxious, and crumbling inside from the lack of care I was receiving. We are often so programmed for external achievement and perfection that we hide our pain from others. Being rewarded for doing the most while you are silently struggling is another way the systems at large continue to strip us of our humanity.

I think this is one of the barriers to rest and energy protection that affect us most often because we tend to be rewarded for our exhaustion. It has taken me years to come to this conclusion. Being brave enough to take up space and center rest and energy conservation daily is a tender practice. I think one of the first steps to making this tangible is realizing that the constant states of depletion we exist in are not normal, no matter what anyone wants us to believe. We can choose more rested versions of ourselves not *just* so we can have more energy to show up for others but so we can feel the presence of peace, aliveness, and groundedness in our own lives. Can you trust that your evolution and growth are still happening, even in your moments of stillness?

Lately, in my trauma-informed workshops and classes, I have been asking folks: Does the presence of rest in your life feel restorative or does it feel like collapse? To me, feeling seen facilitates rest. So much of the work I do as a trauma-informed educator, speaker, and yoga teacher is creating and cultivating spaces where people feel safe enough to rest and know that their choices are celebrated. The stillness of rest reveals so much. The yawns, the tears, and the sighs are all ways the nervous system communicates with us. I find that a lot of the emotions that surface in these workshops comes when participants realize just how exhausted they actually are. The cumulative impact of our exhaustion is so real and valid. You are worthy of spaces where you can practice consent and agency with your own body and where you can slowly unpack what rest means for you. Rest is a deeply personal experience, and each of us is navigating our unique and evolving relationship with it.

My hope is that the frameworks and practices you learn here can be practiced in micro-moments and in ways that feel attainable.

It doesn't have to be a complete overhaul. Instead, you might start by drawing awareness to where you can open up some pockets of time to restore and, most importantly, pour back into yourself. Whether it's closing your eyes for a few moments instead of reaching for your phone to scroll or sitting down to stare out the window and feel the sun on your face instead of completing another task. Over time and with repetition, these new patterns will soften your overstimulation and help you reclaim time that may have otherwise felt unattainable.

Types of Rest Your Nervous System May Be Craving

On her Instagram page, the somatic experiencing expert and practitioner Lexy Florentina shares, "You know you're healing when your palate no longer follows urgency, busyness, and intensity and instead craves slowness, rest, and softness."[7] So much of healing the nervous system is doing the internal work of adopting a slower pace and bravely acknowledging that urgency is not the only way. In this next section, we will get more practical about how you can integrate rest into your life more seamlessly instead of seeing it as something you do only after you have done all of the things.

Many of us may only think of rest as sleep, but there are so many different types of rest that our nervous systems need. The internal medicine physician and work-life integration researcher Dr. Saundra Dalton-Smith offers a framework for the seven types of rest we need—physical, mental, emotional, social, sensory, creative, and spiritual—providing us with a new lens for the way we can tailor the types of support we need amid the seasons we are navigating and the various rest deficits that might be present.[8] The goal is to view these types of rest through the lens of self-care as opposed to "after care," which is a pattern I imagine many of us find ourselves in (taking care of ourselves only after we have reached the point of exhaustion). This makes it hard for rest to ever feel restorative because we are operating from a place of depletion with few reserves to draw from.

You are worthy of resting before you are exhausted.

You are worthy of resting before you are exhausted.

You are worthy of resting before you are exhausted.

Drawing upon Dalton-Smith's framework, I have provided some in-depth examples of how you can engage with particular dimensions of rest in your life and honor what your nervous system is craving. Take your time with this, grab your journal, and let's explore some more restful ways of being.

PHYSICAL REST

Physical rest can be either *passive* or *active*. Passive physical rest includes practices where you are experiencing deep rest and receiving with little output, like sleeping, napping, doing a restorative Yoga Nidra, listening to a sleep meditation or podcast, getting acupuncture or a massage, taking a supported Savasana in the middle of the day, or attending a sound healing class. Active physical rest includes activities that require your participation but are restorative in nature such as yoga, stretching, reading on the couch with a cozy blanket, walking in nature, or any other movement that feels accessible and nourishing to you.

Tending to your basic needs (such as using the restroom or eating when you need to) is also an example of physical rest. At a recent workshop, I asked a group of Montessori teachers if they use the bathroom during the school day, and they gave me the nervous "of course not" laughter. Sometimes honoring physical rest can begin with listening to our bodies and responding with kindness. Physical rest could also look like prioritizing doctor appointments you've been putting off (your mammogram, finding a therapist, the symptom you keep ignoring), practicing preventative self-care, or simply not rushing throughout your day. Let's practice doing that workout, driving to that outing, or even shopping for groceries *real slow*. Instead of trying to carry five grocery bags in from the car, try taking your time to lighten the load (literally and figuratively) or asking for help.

One shift that I introduced you to in the opening of the book is to explore managing your *energy* instead of your *time*. I know it seems like a simple shift, but when energy and bandwidth conservation and mental health become the center, we can really start to see some tangible shifts. For example, you might have time to run errands, but do you have the capacity? I know we don't always have the luxury to ask ourselves these questions because there are people depending on us, but I invite you to integrate this question more regularly into your life so you can make intentional choices that center and honor your well-being.

EMOTIONAL REST

The dimension of emotional rest asks us to reflect on who we are at our core outside of always being there for everyone else. We often spend so much time prioritizing and attuning to the needs of others that we easily neglect our own. If you are a people pleaser or if you struggle to communicate your boundaries at the expense of your well-being, emotional rest may be what you need.

Emotional rest involves creating intentional time for yourself, whether that's being consistent with therapy appointments, asking for help with a specific task, carving out space each day to prioritize and nurture your well-being, cuddling with a pet or loved one, or getting more comfortable with not giving away all of yourself during the day. It takes time, intention, and thoughtfulness to be proactive about your care—but what could be more important?

Other forms of emotional rest could include incorporating a self-care routine upon waking, rescheduling or canceling activities when you are feeling overwhelmed, building mental health days into your calendar, or reclaiming time for yourself to just be.

MENTAL REST

Mental rest takes us back to the beginning of the book when we discussed the cumulative toll of always holding the default nervous system in the room and the tremendous wear and tear this can create. Mental rest is allowing yourself space from constant tasking and saying no without explanation. It could look like building in extra space between meetings and appointments so you have time to downregulate, taking moments to pause and be mindful of when you are overextending yourself and choosing a different way, making space in your day for journaling and stillness, shutting down your devices to reduce the noise of the world, or lowering expectations of yourself and remembering that you do not need to hold it together all of the time. One of the most impactful forms of mental rest is giving yourself permission to unravel and simply be with your feelings just as they are.

CREATIVE REST

In all of my trauma-informed workshops, I find that creative rest seems to be the one folks are most in need of. Creative rest helps reawaken that sense of awe and wonder that lives inside each of us and reignite our spirit in beautiful and expansive ways. This type of rest invites you to immerse yourself in spaces that spark that for you, whether it is nature, your home, a studio, or anywhere else you draw inspiration from. Creative rest helps you reconnect to what you are most passionate about and could involve finding the glimmers and micro-moments of joy throughout your day and viewing things through a new lens. You can begin opening yourself up to creative rest by starting or reengaging with hobbies that make you smile, such as roller skating, karaoke, pottery, painting, or even fashion design. Whatever exercises your creative muscles and puts your mind at ease is perfect!

SPIRITUAL REST

Spiritual rest comes when you're able to connect to something deeply profound and find connection to community, belonging, and a felt sense of purpose and compassion. Spirituality is so personal; it can be dreamed and imagined outside the box and of course will look a little different for each of us. When I think about all of the ways burnout, trauma, and chronic stress have overwhelmed my nervous system and chipped away at my spirit, I realize it was spiritual rest that reignited my light.

Spiritual rest is like a love letter to yourself and a path to recon-necting your pieces. It could involve committing to a restorative daily ritual and routine, connecting to a faith-based community, praying, meditating, engaging in contemplative practices, spending time in nature, listening to a restorative or spiritual playlist (hello India Arie and Beautiful Chorus), setting boundaries with people who deplete you, and avoiding activities that drain your spirit. I don't think we talk enough about the value of protecting our spirits. They deserve our attention and care too.

SENSORY REST

I imagine many of us know overstimulation well: bright lights, computer screens, unlimited scrolling, a barrage of news and information at our fingertips, constant exposure to vicarious trauma, incessant background noise, constant notifications, multitasking, and working far beyond the threshold of what our nervous systems can hold, just to name a few.

All of this can, of course, cause sensory overload and overwhelm. You are human! This can be countered with some much-needed intentional sensory rest. Perhaps you could close your eyes for several minutes in the middle of the day or intentionally unplug at a certain time each day. Similar to the way burnout is sneaky, electronic over-whelm accumulates even when we think we might just be scrolling to relax. We are absorbing so much of the media we consume, and it absolutely impacts our energy. Sensory rest could also look like:

- Using an eye pillow or weighted blanket
- Scheduling alone time to decompress
- Using fidget toys to help soothe your anxiety
- Taking plenty of movement breaks and intentional moments of sensory deprivation
- Practicing the power of repetition, ritual, routine, and consistency
- Putting on soft and comfortable clothes
- Paying attention to your internal body cues when you have reached your threshold and building in a transition/break,

such as closing your laptop, washing your face, doing a brief guided meditation, going for a walk, stepping on the grass, letting the sun touch your body, etc.
- Sitting in silence for a few moments
- Drinking a warm beverage and letting your gaze drift

SOCIAL REST

Sometimes social rest means doing the hard internal work of differentiating between relationships that uplift us and drain us. You deserve to prioritize relationships with people in your life who bring your nervous system a sense of ease. Social rest can look like letting yourself receive a compliment instead of immediately deflecting it, allowing your whole system to relax around supportive friends, leaving texts unread until you have more energy to respond, declining a social request when you are low on capacity, or prioritizing a fun activity with people who fill your cup.

If you need a recap of this section, feel free to refer to the Types of Rest worksheet located in the "Additional Resources" section in the back of the book.

Building Your Rest Inventory

I invite you now to spend some time in reflection with each of these dimensions of rest. If it feels supportive, you can use the examples I provided as prompts, but I encourage you to identify specific examples within each category that are tailored to your unique and nuanced needs. There are no right or wrong answers. By designing your rest inventory, you can begin to make a plan to prioritize more restful experiences into your life.

So much of healing the nervous system is truly learning how to do everything slower and more mindfully. I find that some of my best, most creative ideas and profound teachings come to me when I am taking a long bath, leisurely playing with LEGOs with my son or reading to my daughter, sipping my morning coffee at the table, going on a walk with my dog, engaging in a deep conversation with a beloved friend, resting in a post-meditation practice, laughing about something with my partner, or getting lost in deep presence.

As you start to adopt the frameworks of rest in your life, you might start to notice the gentle shifts that can come with being consistent. Perhaps you'll notice that you're more comfortable with silence, you reach for a book instead of your phone during downtime, you feel more present and connected to your beloveds, or it's easier to find more pockets of energy and joy as you flow through your day. These shifts may seem small, but they are the deeply significant gifts that rest provides us.

GENTLE REMINDER

Healing can reveal itself in many subtle ways. From coffee with a friend, a nature walk, a yoga class, or a sweet interaction with a stranger. May you never underestimate the moments of living that are healing, restorative, and replenishing to your spirit and your light. Sometimes the most beautiful lessons arrive without you striving for them.

Affirmations for Rest

The following rest affirmations can be woven throughout your day in moments you need them most. They can be recited quietly in your head or spoken aloud in front of a mirror. I hope they provide soft landings, an inner sanctuary, and space for you to reimagine and reclaim your tenderness.

- I exist in all the soft and sacred moments where I can take my armor off and rest.
- I lean into and reimagine my softness.
- I deserve a slower and softer pace of life.
- Prioritizing rest is integral to my healing.

- I deserve so much more than constant cycles of depletion and burnout.
- I offer myself grace when overwhelm, stress, pressure, and burnout start to sink in.
- I am worthy even when I don't overextend myself.
- I am in charge of protecting my peace.
- I release what no longer aligns to create space for all parts of me to be free.
- It's okay to release the pressure of being resilient all the time. Sometimes resilience looks like rest.
- I prioritize myself first.
- Rest is inherently mine.
- My softness and sensitivity are my most powerful forms of strength.
- I am worthy of easing the amount of pressure and burden I place on myself.
- I freely let myself unravel and feel.
- I open myself up to the joy and comfort of being fully seen.
- Ease is available to me.
- I am so deserving of the presence of peace in my life.
- I am worthy of honoring my changing capacity.
- I make space today to find my inner sanctuary.
- Today and every day I anchor myself in the rituals and routines that settle my nervous system.
- I courageously ask for tangible support.
- Sleep might just be the answer today.
- I don't have to overexplain myself.
- I deserve the compassion I so freely give and pour into others.
- In every season of life, I water the parts of me that need tending.
- I don't have to compartmentalize my feelings. All parts of my experience are welcome.
- I celebrate my beautiful heart while also honoring my boundaries as sacred.
- Tenderness is my love language.
- In every season of life, I honor and celebrate all versions of myself.

- I am worthy of taking up all of the space I deserve.
- I honor the people and spaces that support the health of my nervous system.
- I live slowly. I take all the time I need.
- I tend to my overwhelm with mindfulness, intention, and care.
- I celebrate all the sacred moments I choose rest over productivity.
- I release shame and guilt; they do not belong in my heart.
- Today and every day, I offer myself more patience and grace amid everything I am holding.
- I consciously and intentionally choose to do less.
- I am beautiful and enough just as I am.
- I celebrate the seemingly simple and sacred moments of my life.
- I deserve help with the mental load I carry. I don't have to do this alone.
- I am worthy of tending to my mental health with care.
- I take time to do what replenishes my spirit.
- I am worthy of receiving help and support.
- I nurture what feels affirming and life-giving.
- I do the work to cultivate my joy.
- I deserve to pause and pace myself.
- I am worthy of soft landings.

Trauma-Informed Yoga Shapes to Explore When You're Exhausted

In this section I invite you to engage with my personal rest tool kit, which includes some of my favorite trauma-informed yoga shapes of rest. Trauma-informed yoga is an evidence-based healing modality and an empowering yoga practice that prioritizes the lived experiences and healing of each student. Safety, trust, choice, and agency are some of the core components that guide the practice. If you only have five minutes to spare in your day, I encourage you to explore the shapes that are accessible to you to help nurture and reset your nervous system.

Trauma-informed yoga can support you with building vagal tone and enhancing your overall health, well-being, and resilience. The practice helps to widen your window of tolerance, build nervous system flexibility, and strengthen your coping skills. It is a practice that can support the activation of your parasympathetic (relaxed) nervous system and create more space for safety, rest, growth, and joy. Additional benefits of a trauma-informed yoga practice include:

- Recognition of choice in one's life
- Ability to be more expressive in therapy
- Decreased feelings of depression, stress, and anxiety
- Increased confidence and courage
- Increased feelings of self-compassion
- Increased awareness of needs, mindfulness skills, and resiliency
- Strengthened self-esteem
- Strengthened emotional, physical, mental, spiritual, and interpersonal skills
- Increased feelings of being seen, valued, and affirmed[9]

RECOMMENDED PROPS

Here are a few props that can support you in these shapes; however, these are optional. Feel free to modify and drop into these shapes even if you have limited props available.

- Yoga mat
- Bolster or pillow
- Meditation cushion
- Blocks
- Blanket
- Eye pillow
- Cozy socks
- Water bottle
- Journal

SETTING UP YOUR SPACE

As you start to set up your space, you might envision that you are creating a sanctuary—a soft place to land—for someone you love and cherish. You could lay out a yoga mat and have a bolster, blanket, and blocks nearby to hold and support you as you move through the shapes. Feel free to play restorative music and have a warm beverage on hand. Cultivate a space where you can be gentle with yourself, whatever that looks like for you.

LEGS UP THE WALL POSE (VIPARITA KARANI)

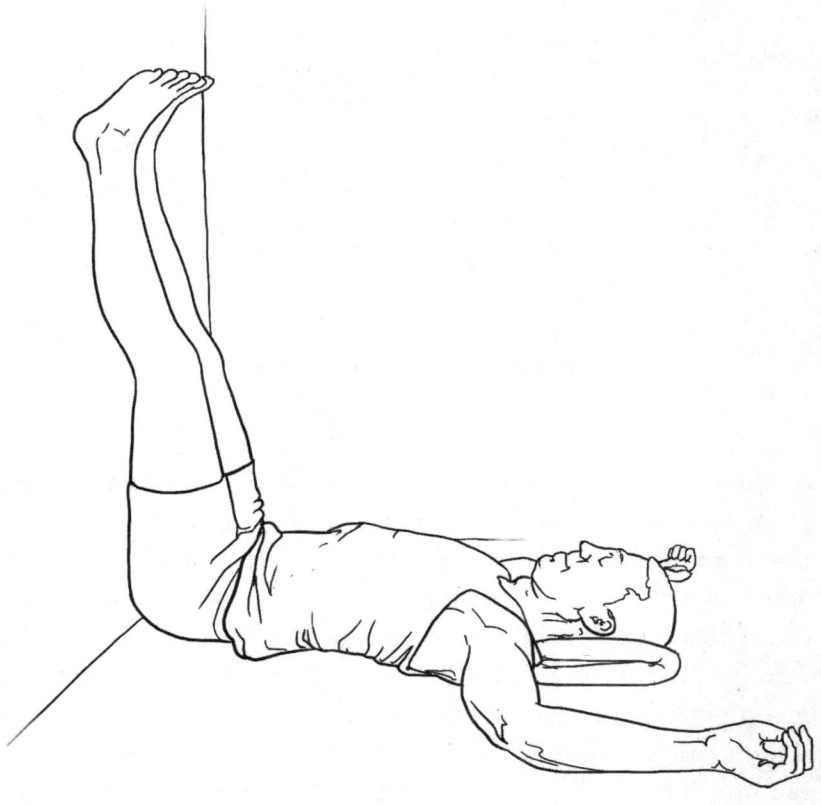

Legs Up the Wall Pose (Viparita Karani) helps
stimulate our body's relaxation response.

If it feels supportive and accessible to you, explore lying on your back
and drawing your legs up a solid wall. You might prefer a variation of
this shape by resting your legs on a couch or chair. Find any shape that
invites feelings of restoration, allows you to feel held, and honors the
support and care of the earth beneath you. Take your time to linger in
the magic of this moment. Let your body soak in the benefits of this
parasympathetic nervous system activation.

SUPPORTED CORPSE POSE (SAVASANA)

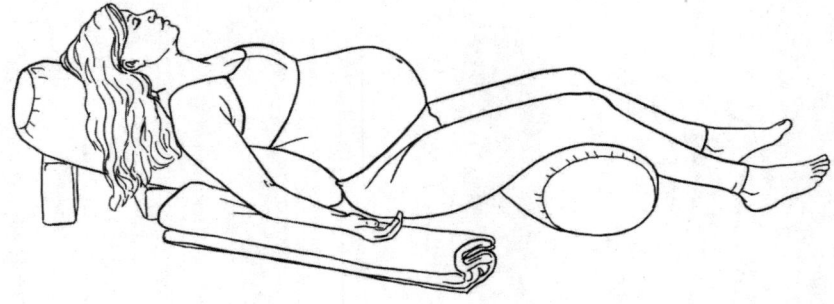

Supported Savasana helps promote deep rest.

Your Savasana is yours, and you are always supported and encouraged to find your own unique shape of rest. On your inhale, hug your body in gratitude and trust the strength of your body to hold you. Honor yourself and your practice, and on your exhale, explore a final resting posture that feels comfortable in your body. There is no exact way to rest, so find a shape that helps you feel safe and supported. For a supported Savasana, you can first explore bringing one block vertical to the back of your mat and one block horizontal a few inches in front of it. Then place a bolster or blanket over the blocks and gently rest your back into the support of these props. For extra support, you might bring another bolster or blanket underneath your knees, and roll up blankets and place them underneath your arms. If you have an eye pillow, this might be the perfect time to use it! As displayed in the image, feel free to explore using any props available to you to allow your body to feel held and supported. Please also feel welcome to explore lying on your side or stay seated if that feels better for you. You can also place your hands on your belly to focus on your mindful breathing.

Take a scan of your body, finding an anchor and connecting to the energy of the earth beneath you. Rest in this space of listening to what your body needs. Allow the sensations of your body to meet the strength of your breath.

RECLINING TWIST POSE (SUPTA MATSYENDRASANA)

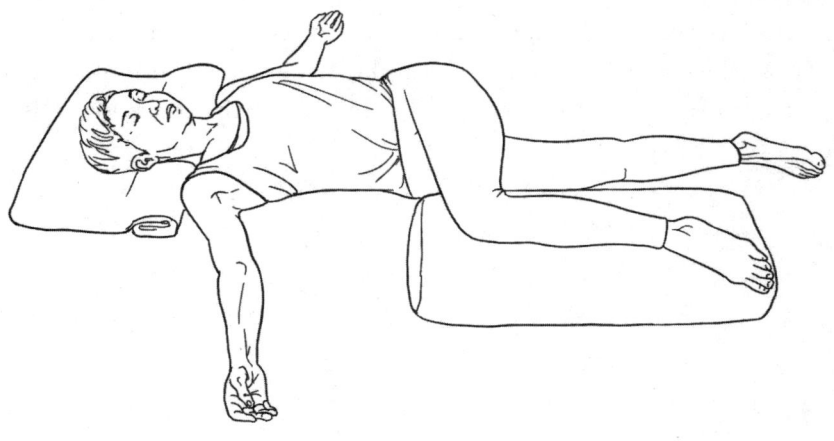

Reclining Twist Pose (Supta Matsyendrasana)
invites you to unwind and release.

Gently lie on your back and hug your knees to your heart. If you'd like, you could circle your knees to the right, almost like you are drawing circles on the ceiling with your knees. Switch sides to the left whenever you feel ready. In your own time and in a way that's accessible to you, hug your knees back into your heart space and explore massaging your sacrum/lower back into your mat. Inhale to hug everything in and exhale, extending your right leg long and letting your left knee fall over to the right side of your body. It might feel good to rest your knee on top of a bolster or blanket for extra support.

On your next inhale, I invite you to notice the length of your spine, and exhale to deepen the stretch to a degree that feels available to you. Rest here for as long as you'd like. Allow your body to melt with each exhale. On your next inhale, hug your knees to your heart once more, and on your next exhale, extend your left leg long and let your right knee fall to the left side of your body. Once again, on your inhale, notice the length of your spine, and as you exhale, deepen the stretch to a degree that feels available to you. Allow your body to linger here for as long as feels good.

When you feel ready, hug everything in, and with so much com-passion and care, make your way up to a seated shape. You might rest a palm over your belly and a palm over your heart to feel the rise and fall of your breath. Allow the warmth of your breath to radiate out with each exhale. Take your time before making the transition to the rest of your day.

SUPPORTED BUTTERFLY POSE (BADDHA KONASANA)

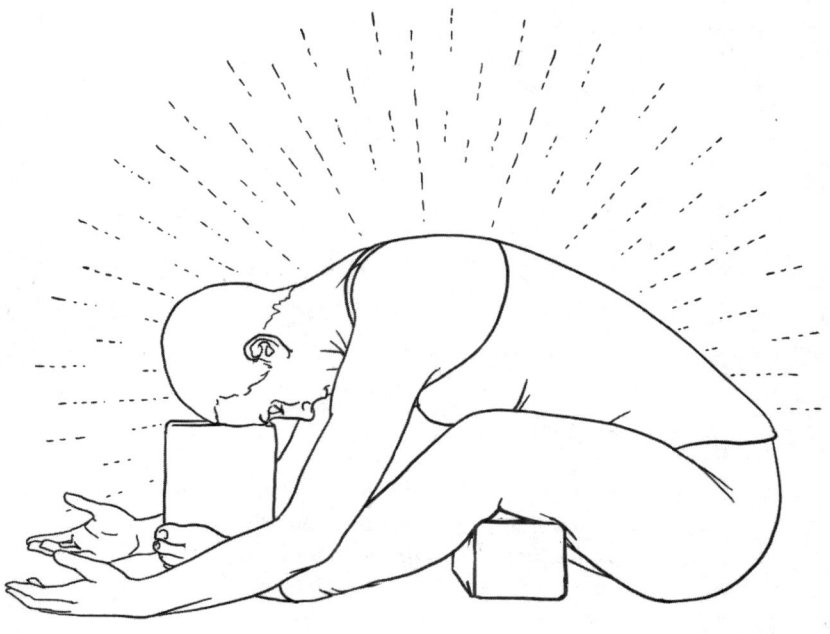

Supported Butterfly Pose (Baddha Konasana)
helps restore the nervous system.

I invite you to gather four blocks to support you in feeling held in this shape. Find a seated shape that feels supportive to your body. If you'd like, you can bring the soles of your feet together and place a block underneath each knee for added support. You might stay here, resting a palm over your heart and a palm over your belly. If you want to explore folding forward from here, you can stack two blocks slightly in front of your feet and gently rest your forehead on the blocks.

Take as much time as you need to make any adjustments and increase your comfort. Allow this to be a sacred time to feel the support of the earth, restore and recalibrate your nervous system, and honor your need for deep rest.

SUPPORTED BRIDGE POSE (SETU BANDHASANA)

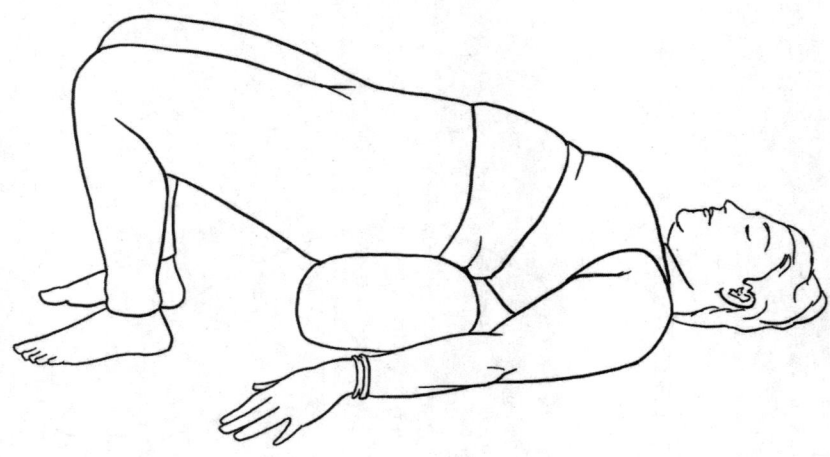

Supported Bridge Pose (Setu Bandhasana)
promotes self-compassion and grace.

If it feels comfortable and accessible for your body, explore resting on your back and drawing the soles of your feet to the mat or ground beneath you. Allow your arms to fall wherever feels comfortable. On your inhale, gently lift your hips and slide a block underneath your sacrum/lower back. On your exhale, allow yourself to melt into the support of the block and know that you are held and lifted. You are never alone in what you are navigating.

Allow your breath to radiate from the base of your spine all the way up to the crown of your head. With each inhale and exhale, allow yourself to release what feels heavy, even if just for a moment, within the container of this space and practice. Give yourself all of the compassion and grace you deserve. Continue in this shape for as long as it feels safe and supportive for you.

SUPPORTED CHILD'S POSE (BALASANA)

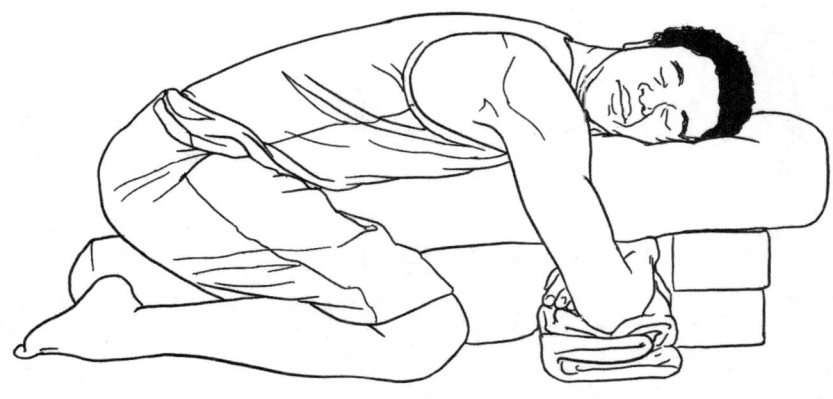

Supported Child's Pose (Balasana) helps you feel
held amid all the holding you do for others.

Rest your bolster or pillow vertically on your mat or on the ground, then make your way into Child's Pose, bringing your knees to the outside edges of your mat and allowing your feet to touch if that feels comfortable. Gently lie on the bolster, resting your cheek and your gaze. You can hug the bolster with your arms and melt a little deeper with each exhale. Feel free to incorporate any additional props to increase your comfort and care. Be so generous and considerate of yourself, love. Take up all of the space you deserve.

SUPPORTED FORWARD FOLD POSE
(PASCHIMOTTANASANA)

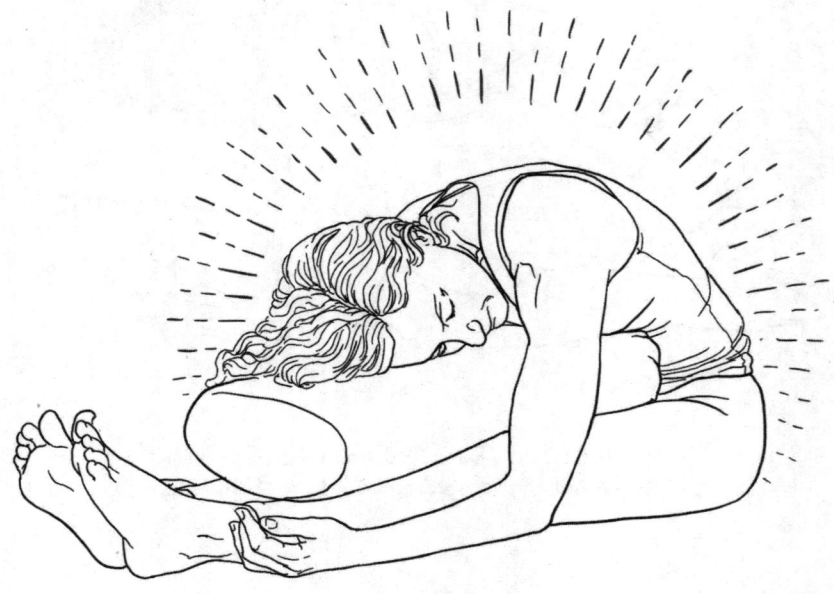

Supported Forward Fold Pose (Paschimottanasana)
allows you to honor your body's needs.

Find a supported, seated shape and gently extend your legs in front of you. You can allow your feet to touch or separate them to create space for your pillow, bolster, or blocks. If you decide to use one, rest your pillow or bolster over your legs and gently lie your body over the prop. Or if it feels more supportive, you can stack your blocks between your knees and rest your forehead on top of the blocks. Take your time to find your sweet, sacred spot and make any adjustments you need. You are worthy of this time to honor and center your needs, tune out the world, and take note of all the ways you are supported. Allow being where you are in this moment to be enough. It is enough.

A Closing Rest Meditation to Support the Cultivation of Ease and Tenderness

This meditation can be used to support you in cultivating more ease, gentleness, and tenderness in your day. Feel free to practice this whenever you are feeling overwhelmed or simply need respite from the hustle and bustle of your schedule.

To begin, I invite you to gently settle in a way that feels right to you and notice what holds you here today. Know that you deserve to feel held and supported amid all of the holding that you do. Take a sacred pause here; maybe a deeper, braver breath. This is a moment to ground and just be. For a moment, allow everything that you've been carrying to roll off of your shoulders and onto the safety of the space beneath you. On your inhale, gently draw your shoulders up, and on your exhale, relax them back and down your spine. Offer yourself gratitude for arriving, for carving out this time, for reminding yourself that your needs matter.

As you soften and relax, you might start to notice where you feel ease or constriction. Know that whatever is present for you is welcome. Take a moment here to make a shift or a change, moving your body or reaching for an extra prop as needed. You can reach for an extra blanket or a pillow, a bolster for underneath your knees, or anything that allows you to melt into the space beneath you. Continue to engage with your breath in a way that feels nurturing. You don't have to earn your rest.

You're welcome to keep your eyes closed or open, maybe finding a soft gaze in front of you. Choose what feels most supportive in your body. Let your breath rest here. Trust the strength of your body to hold you here. Notice the subtle rise and fall of your breath.

In this renewed space of rest, try to follow the wave of energy that radiates from the base of your spine all the way up to your heart space. If you'd like, you can even rest your palms over your heart and connect to your beautiful, powerful breath.

If it feels right, you can set an intention for this practice, something that allows you to connect deeply to what rest means for you or acknowledge the rest you might be craving. Allow yourself to lean into the fullness of this experience. You could reflect on an affirmation, a mantra, or a safe visualization of a place that immerses you in a space of ease. Anything that supports you with orienting back to your body. If at any time your bodily sensations feel too overwhelming, bring your focus back to this intention or something outside of your body, such as the nature outside of your window or a pet that's sharing your space.

Now I invite you to anchor into the support beneath you, whether that is your mat, a cushion, or the ground. Take note of what it feels like to be held and supported. Gently tune in to your breath once again and find a pace that gently supports you. There's no need to control your breathing in any way. Notice whatever arises for you here, knowing that there is space for all of it. To tend and to hold. To be reminded that you're not alone. To remember that it's not your fault if rest is difficult for you.

Take a deep, full inhale to honor your intention, then with an open mouth, exhale and melt a little bit deeper into the space beneath you. If it's available to you, using both hands, make peace signs with your fingers and gently ground your fingertips into the mat or cushion beneath you. This is called Bhu Mudra. Breathe here in this space, releasing any burdens with each exhale. Honor a few moments of silence to access the depth of your breath and presence.

When you are ready, make your way to a final Savasana, or resting shape. Know that you're welcome to stay in any shape that honors your body. You could explore lying on your belly, on your side, on your back with knees to your heart, or perhaps a seated meditation or Legs Up the Wall Pose. You could even grab additional props for more support. Your rest is yours. Once you're comfortable, feel free to stay in this space of deep relaxation for as long as you'd like.

When you feel ready, invite a little bit of movement back into your body. Wiggle your toes and fingers, circle your ankles or wrists— whatever is accessible to you. You could even interlace your fingers and stretch your arms overhead, finding the length from the base of your spine all the way up through the crown of your head.

As you meet the rest of your day, remember to honor your cues of exhaustion and trust yourself and your needs. Recognize when it's time to turn down the chatter of the outside world and return to yourself. Be discerning with what you say yes to. Leave the dishes in the sink, the laundry in the baskets, the toys on the floor. Find frequent moments to sit down, rest your gaze, and simply listen to the sound of your breath. Remind yourself often that you may not get to everything on your list, and that's okay.

As we close out this meditation, reflect on how these reminders landed for you. Be gentle and kind to your mind, reflecting on the intention or mantra that guided your practice today. Meet me with your palms together at the center of your heart or find any other expression that feels supportive. Hands at your heart, may we live our lives compassionately. Hands at your mouth, may we speak words of truth and kindness. Hands at your third-eye center, the light in me always honors the light in you. May the divine always guide your way. Namaste.

This meditation presented a lot of inquiries and points of reflection, so if you have space today, I encourage you to journal about whatever might have come up for you. I'm sending you so much care, love, and compassion and wishing you deep rest.

To access an audio recording of this meditation,
visit us.macmillan.com/ProtectYourEnergy.

. . . .

I hope this chapter has helped you begin to reconceptualize the role of rest in your life. I hope your spirit feels reinvigorated and that you are inspired with new ideas and practices for restoring your nervous system and finding more ease. There is so much space to be found in reclaiming the seemingly ordinary but sacred moments of our lives.

The final chapter of this book is overflowing with more micro self-care practices you can add to your tool kit to widen your window of tolerance; find your sweet and sacred spot; tend to your energy with intention, compassion, and grace; and continue your journey of nurturing a flexible and resilient nervous system.

7

Micro Self-Care Practices and Trauma-Informed Meditations to Protect Your Energy

> You did all of that with weight on your
> wings. I can't wait to see you flying free.[1]
> —DR. THEMA BRYANT

In this final chapter, I will introduce you to a variety of embodied micro self-care practices that you can weave into your daily life. Explore these practices at your pace and integrate into your tool kit only what resonates with you. You can also revisit the Assessing Your Energy worksheet in the "Additional Resources" section to get a sense of the most depleting activities in your life and, wherever possible, begin to swap in some of these practices for healing, stress relief, restoration, or support. Make it a habit to honor what you need each day instead of just focusing on what needs to get done. May these practices be a reminder that you are a priority in your own life.

Trauma-Informed Practices for Releasing Tension Stored in the Nervous System

Feel free to reference the following list for ideas of what nervous system practices to engage in during particular emotional moments.

Each of these will be detailed within the chapter and can serve as a guide when you are in need of self-compassion, grounding, healing, safety, calm and peace, boundaries, a nervous system reset, joy, rest, and release. These practices are not meant to be prescriptive and can of course be used interchangeably, but when we are overwhelmed, it can be nice to have something to reference. As always, integrate what resonates and feel free to modify these practices to make them more accessible for you.

- **When in need of self-compassion and safety**, try a butterfly hug and rocking yourself, five-step self-holding, embodied self-compassion practice, or face cradle.
- **When in need of grounding**, try earthing, resourcing, and grounding techniques.
- **When in need of calm and peace**, try a walking meditation, visualizing a calm place, or resting with support of props.
- **When in need of boundaries**, try an energy protection meditation or Warrior I release.
- **When in need of a nervous system reset**, try a seated meditation with self-massage, inner light meditation, or heart and ear soothing.
- **When in need of release**, try a sun meditation to thaw grief, stress, and tension; Chair Pose (Utkatasana) to release self-doubt; or a Ragdoll release.
- **When in need of healing and joy**, try an expand-and-contract exercise, either by spending time in nature or with a gentle head cradle and heart opening.

BUTTERFLY HUG AND ROCKING YOURSELF

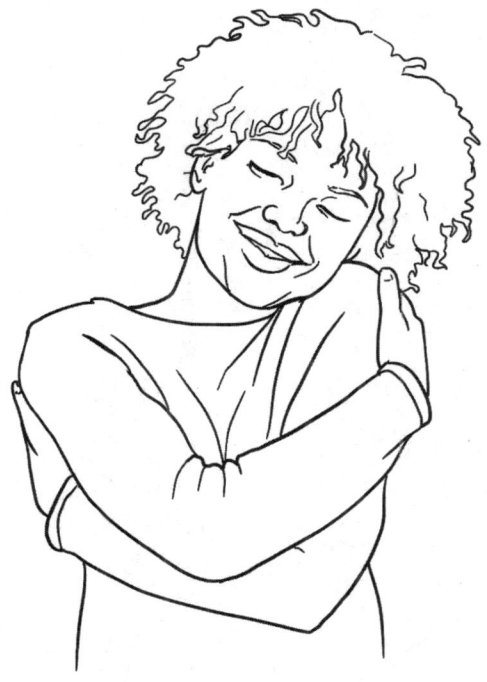

Giving yourself a butterfly hug is a great way to
offer yourself support and compassion.

Take a moment to find a comfortable seated shape. If it feels right,
cross your arms over your chest and rest the right side of your cheek
on top of your left palm and offer yourself a supportive, warm, and
compassionate hug. If it feels okay to continue, you can explore
switching sides and rest your left cheek on top of your right palm.
Feel free to integrate a gentle rocking movement if that feels good for
you. Stay here for as long as you'd like. Take all the time you need
to linger in your own care; there is no rush. This is your body, your
practice, and always your choice.

SUN MEDITATION

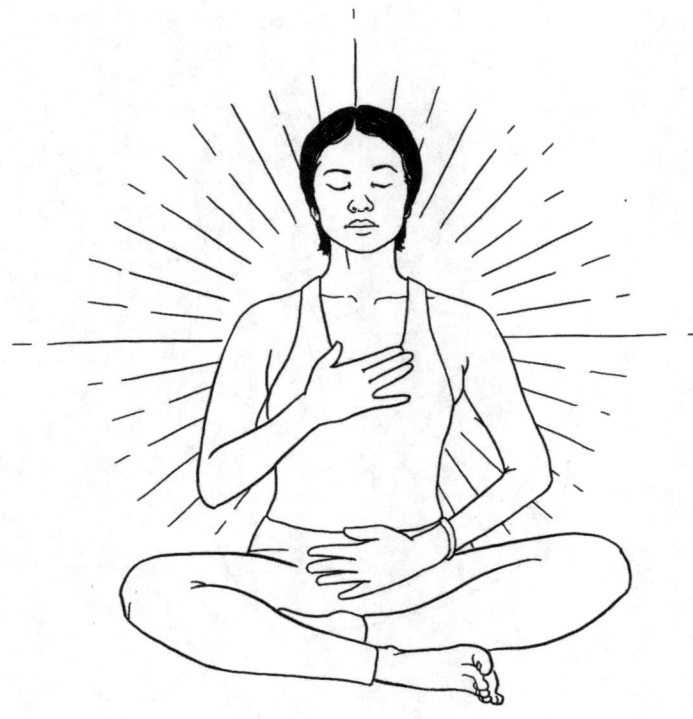

Sun meditation can help you thaw grief, trauma, stress,
and tension that might be present in your body.

I invite you to find a comfortable shape outside or inside by a window. Release your shoulders down and back and place your attention on the feeling of the sun on any parts of your body that need extra care and support. You could even envision that the sun is softening and thawing any areas of your body that are holding grief, trauma, stress, or tension. Explore turning the volume of your heart all the way up and the volume of your thoughts all the way down. Notice where you might feel even a small sense of softening. Just as the sun helps to thaw grief, stress, or tension, it is also an energy source. Allow this moment to revive you and give you strength. You are doing an amazing job.

SEATED MEDITATION AND SELF-MASSAGE

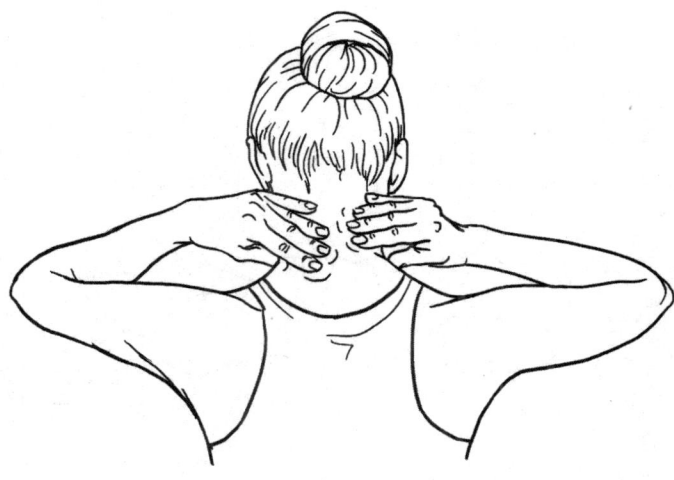

A seated meditation and self-massage practice can
help reorient you back to your body's needs.

Begin in any seated position that feels supportive to your body—
perhaps on a mat, bolster, blanket, or chair. Bring one hand to your
belly and one hand to your heart. In this space, take a moment to
notice the rise and fall of your breath. If being with this internal
sensation feels too overwhelming, focus on something external in
the room, outside of your body—perhaps a color, a sound, or another
resource. Choose what feels soothing and supports you in safely reorienting back to your body.

If it feels supportive and accessible, bring your palms to the back
of your shoulders and offer yourself a gentle self-massage. Bring this
level of awareness and attention to any other parts of your body that
need care and support right now, like your face, temples, earlobes,
neck, the back of your head, or forearms. Offer yourself tenderness,
compassion, and attention in this way for as long as you'd like.

RESTING WITH THE SUPPORT OF PROPS

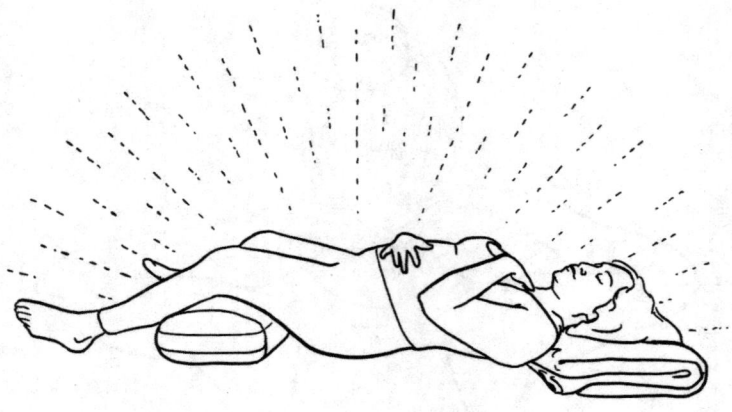

Allow the props to support you amid all
of the holding you do for others.

If you notice you are in need of sensory self-care, take a moment
to turn off all devices, dim the lights if that feels okay for you, and
reach for any props to support you, like pillows, bolsters, blankets,
or an eye pillow. Set up your space in a way that feels nourishing
and abundant. As you gently ground into your space, know that you
are worthy of support. Take as much time as you need to find your
unique shape of rest. Notice what it feels like to be held amid all
of the holding you do for others. You are worthy of your own care.
Take a moment to send yourself gratitude for carving out this time
for yourself. So often that is the hardest part.

VISUALIZE A CALM PLACE

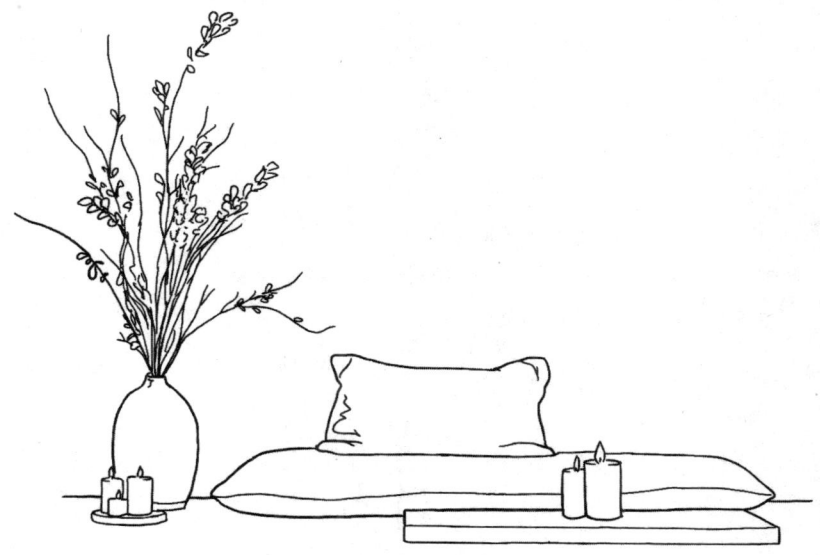

Anchor yourself and connect to your
joy by visualizing a calm place.

If you find yourself moving quickly throughout your day and feeling overwhelmed, take a few moments to cultivate a nourishing place of stillness and ease. If you would like, rest a palm on your heart and a palm on your belly and connect with the rise and fall of your breath. Take as much time as you need to gently settle in and begin to bring to mind a place that brings you a sense of calm, peace, and ease. It might be somewhere you have visited, or it might be a place you create in your mind. Allow yourself to take in the full senses of that place, perhaps even letting your shoulders relax down your spine as you ground into the energy and beauty of it all. Come back to this place any time you need to connect to your joy and settle your nervous system.

WALKING MEDITATION

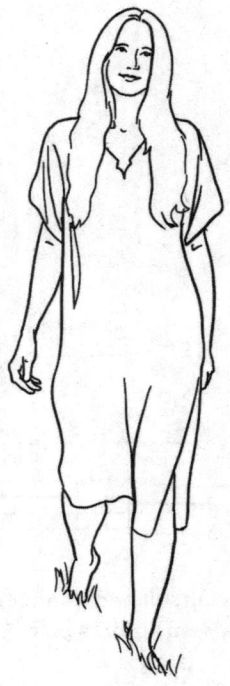

Take your time in walking meditation as you trust
the strength of the earth to hold you.

Sometimes sitting for meditation can feel activating for those who have experienced trauma. If this is you, and if it feels supportive and accessible to you, I invite you to explore taking a meditative walk instead. If you can, leave your devices behind and fully immerse yourself in this experience to engage all of your senses and, most importantly, your attention. Notice the way your feet feel in the grass or on the pavement, connect with the feeling of the breeze and the sun on your face, and take in all of the ways that nature can reset your nervous system and offer feelings of ease and groundedness. There is no need to rush this process. Trust the strength of the earth and your body to hold you here.

RESOURCING

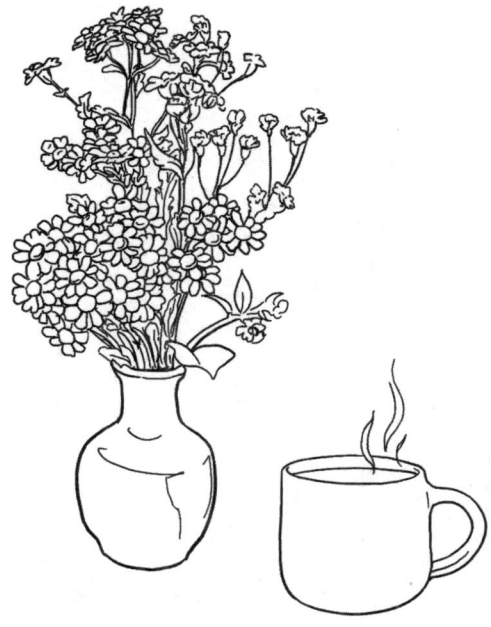

You deserve to find a resource that brings
you peace, comfort, and joy.

As we've learned, resourcing is the act of mindfully identifying a person, place, sound, or thing that generates feelings of well-being, neutrality, peace, comfort, joy, or calm. You might explore this before a meeting or activity that feels either draining or activating, or you may decide to take a moment to return to yourself if you find that you have been overgiving or overextending.

I invite you to take a moment to gaze around your space and take note of anything that brings you a sense of joy and grounding. It might be a pet, a vase of fresh flowers, or a warm cup of coffee. Take in your surroundings with the full senses of your mind, body, and spirit and intentionally honor the messages of your nervous system before launching into whatever might be next on your list. You deserve to take your time.

EMBODIED SELF-COMPASSION
PRACTICE AND FACE CRADLE

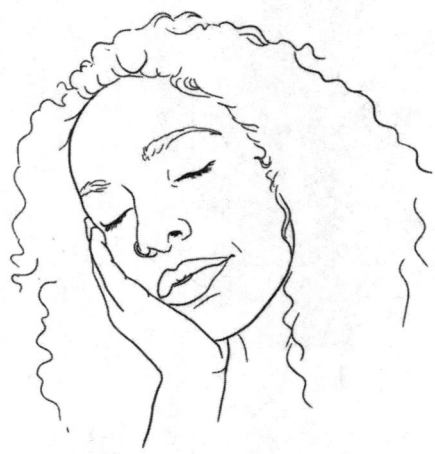

A face cradle practice is a wonderful way to
offer yourself softness and support.

When you feel ready, find a seated shape that offers you a sense of safety and ease. Take all the time you need to set yourself up and use as many props as you need to increase your comfort. Begin by rubbing your palms together and creating a little bit of warmth. Whenever it feels right for you, gently rest your palms over your heart to take in your own care and compassion. Perhaps you'll even feel called to gently rock side to side.

When you are ready, bring your right hand to your right cheek and gently cradle it. Sink a little bit deeper into your palm with each exhale, allowing yourself to feel the comfort of your own support and touch. Can you give yourself permission to take in the tenderness you so freely share with others? Switch sides whenever you would like and bring your left hand to your left cheek and gently cradle it. Take all the time you need here to find grounding in your own worthiness and softness. You are worthy of feeling seen. Allow being where you are to be enough. It is enough.

GROUNDING PRACTICES

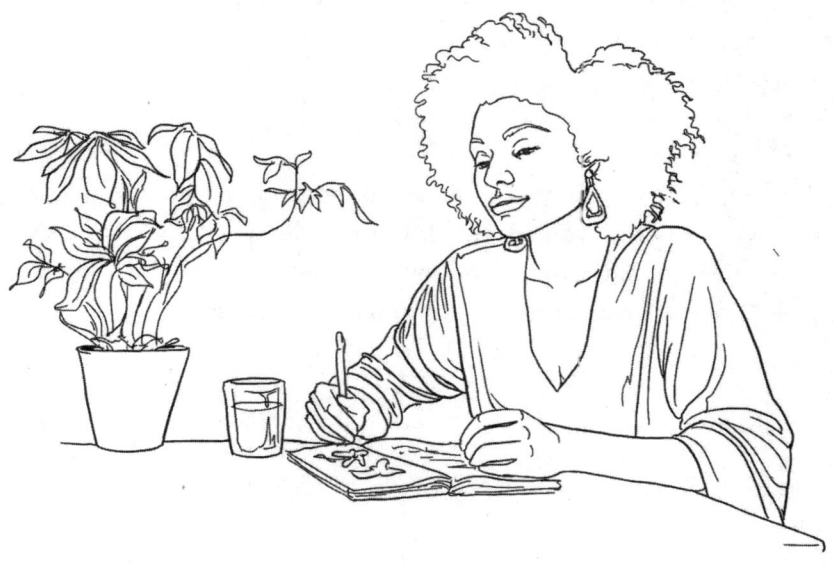

Engage in grounding practices to minimize
stress and center yourself.

Grounding practices can help us feel more balanced by providing moments of calm in the middle of a hectic day. They can help you tend to your inner landscape with gentleness and compassion. Here are just a few examples you might explore:

- Identify one thing in your surroundings that you can see, hear, feel, taste, and smell.
- Hold a grounding object, such as a stone, crystal, or some other tangible object.
- Release anxious feelings with a fidget toy.
- Rest one palm on your heart and one palm on your belly and focus on the rise and fall of your breath.
- Notice the sensation of your feet on the ground or the support of the chair underneath you.

- Integrate mindfulness into all aspects of the day (while in a therapy session, sipping coffee/tea, washing dishes, driving, etc.).
- Drink water.
- Take slow breaths at your pace.
- Journal.
- Anchor in feelings of gratitude by reflecting on one thing in your day that you felt thankful for and that gave you a sense of embodied warmth and joy.
- Cry and give yourself space to feel and release.

EXPAND AND CONTRACT: HEALING AND NATURE

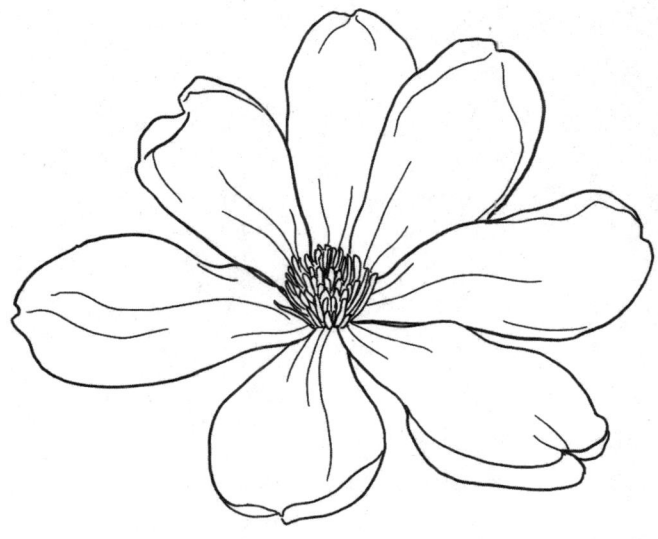

Like the earth, we're constantly moving through
stages of expansion and contraction.

Madison Abdallah, a somatic experiencing professional, shared a
video of a dahlia flower and its natural flow of expansion and contraction.[2] It was such a beautiful reminder of the nonlinear process
of healing and the ways the nervous system is often mirrored in
nature. Just like a flower contracts and expands, wilts and blooms,
so do we. Remind yourself of this in the seasons that feel trying, and
remember that everything is temporary and that we are constantly
evolving.

With this in mind, I invite you to take a deep breath in to embody
this reminder and slowly exhale at your pace, your way. Take some
time today to lean into the grounding and nurturing elements of
nature and notice the inherent, divine connection between your body
and the earth. Your spirit will thank you.

GENTLE HEAD CRADLE WITH HEART OPENING

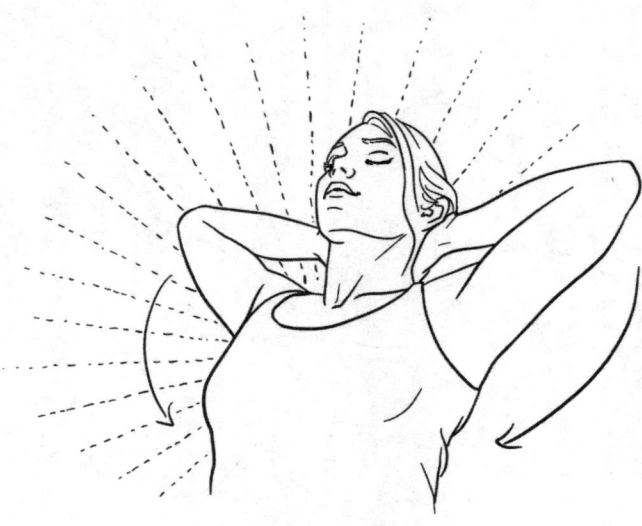

Recenter your energy with a gentle
head cradle and heart opening.

From a seated shape, I invite you to gently interlace your fingers and rest your palms behind your head, drawing your elbows out to a degree that feels comfortable to you. On your inhale, lean back and shine your heart up toward the sky. On your exhale, draw your energy inward like you are cocooning into your body. Again, inhale to lift your heart up to the sky, and exhale to draw everything in. Move through as many rounds of this breath as you'd like to begin shifting and recentering the energy in your body amid whatever you might be carrying and navigating in this moment.

CHAIR POSE (UTKATASANA)

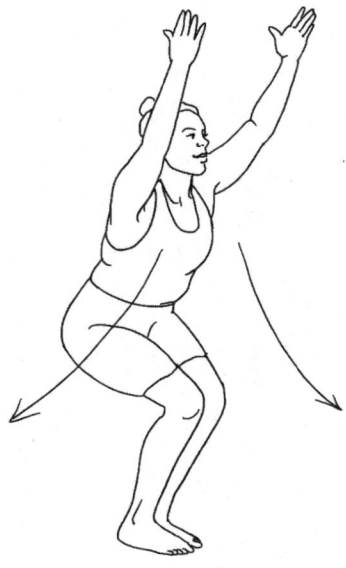

Explore this version of Chair Pose (Utkatasana)
to help you release self-doubt, shame, and guilt.[3]

If it is accessible for you, come to a standing position, bring your feet together, and gently bend your knees like you are sitting in a chair. Bend only as deeply as feels comfortable for you. You can also modify this posture by sitting on a chair and raising your arms above your head. On your inhale, extend your arms high to the sky, and on your exhale, sweep your arms to the right side of your body to release self-doubt, shame, guilt, or any other negative emotions you may be carrying. Inhale to bring your arms back to center, high in the sky, and exhale to sweep your arms to the left side of your body. Repeat this as often as needed to gently shift out energy that does not serve you and release what feels heavy.

INNER LIGHT MEDITATION

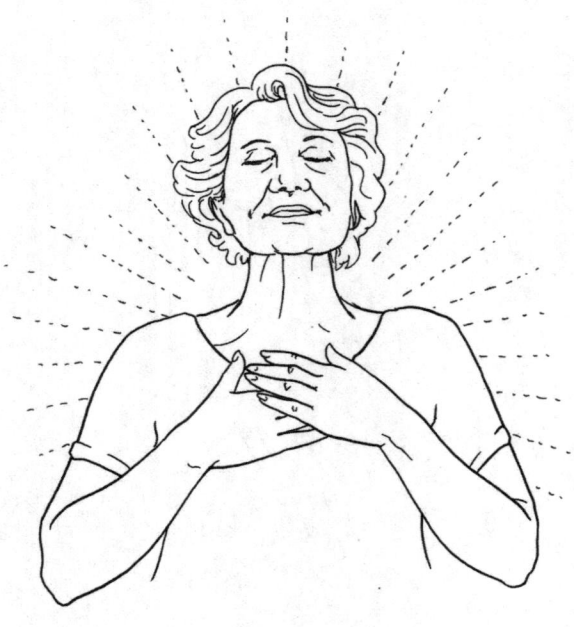

You deserve to bask in your inner light.

Rub your palms together to create a little bit of warmth, then gently rest them on any parts of your body that feel exhausted, depleted, or worn out. Where do you feel that tension in your body? Be intentional here as you practice taking in your own light. Explore crossing your arms across your chest and gently massaging your shoulders, your forearms, and your palms. Invite in a gentle rocking motion if it feels supportive to you. When you are ready, rub your palms together again and then gently rest them over your heart to embody your warmth. You are worth your attention and care.

ENERGY PROTECTION MEDITATION

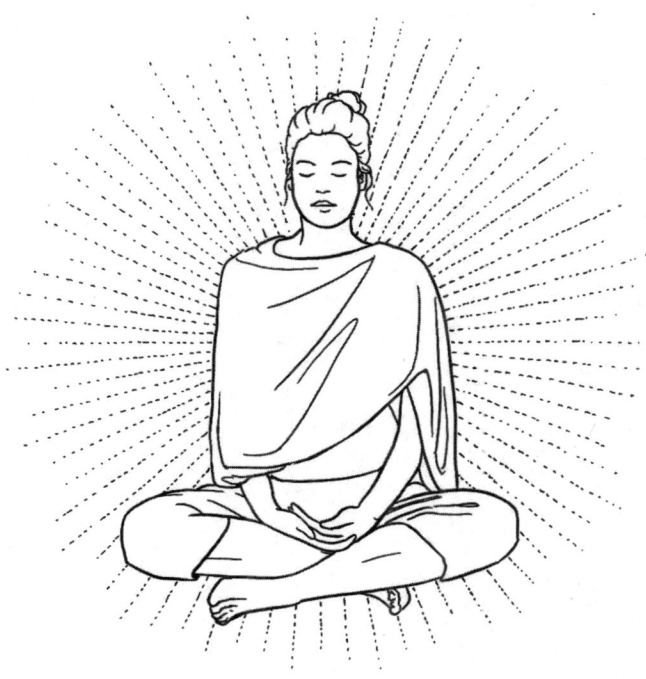

Create a buffer of protection around you with
this energy protection meditation.

If you are feeling like your boundaries are being tested, I invite you
to find any seated shape that feels supportive to you—perhaps sitting
on a chair, a mat, or a cushion with your legs crossed or sitting on
the backs of your heels with your knees together. Feel free to reach
for any props to increase your comfort. Next, imagine that there is
a warm circle of light surrounding you and creating an energetic
boundary. Visualize for a moment that you are circling yourself with
your own energy and light. Envision that this light is radiating out
and creating a buffer of protection around you. You deserve to protect your peace.

HEART AND EAR SOOTHING

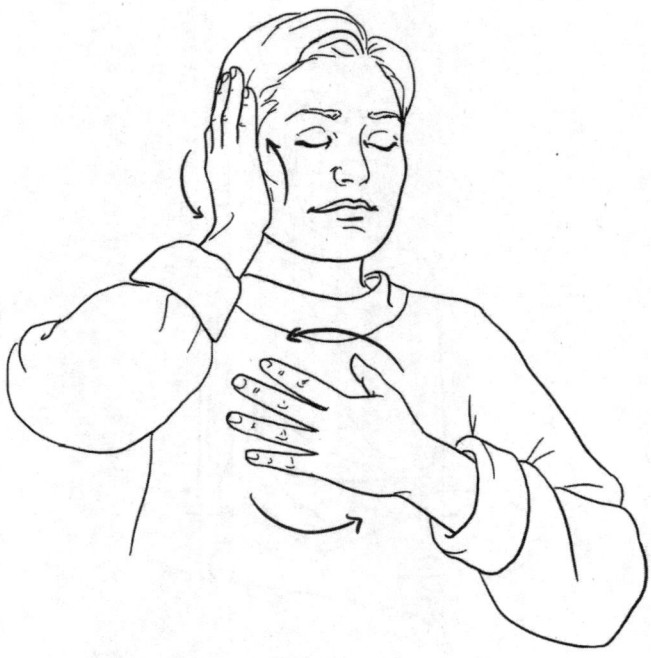

This heart and ear soothing practice invites you
to tend to yourself with intention and care.

If you are working through some difficult emotions, holding grief,
or feeling anxious, I invite you to explore this soothing heart and
ear practice. Find a comfortable shape to begin. Rub your palms
together to create some warmth and explore a gentle and soothing
circular motion with one palm over your heart space and one palm
over your ear. Tune in to the sensations and sounds of this gentle
practice. Allow yourself to get lost in this space of compassion. Feel
free to stay here for as long as feels comfortable. Switch hands whenever you feel ready.

EARTHING

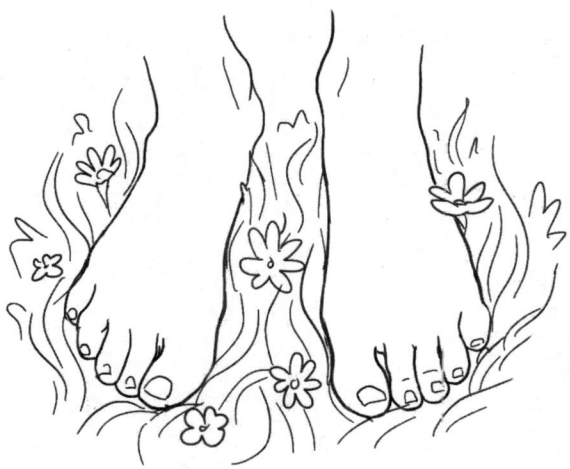

Ground yourself in the present moment
with an earthing practice.

If it feels accessible to you, explore walking barefoot in the grass and allow the soles of your feet to ground into the earth. Take note of the feeling of the sun on your face and the sounds of the birds, the breeze, and any other nature elements that arise. Allow your mind, body, and spirit to take in the totality of the present moment. Take your time here and know that you are worthy of being held, supported, and nurtured by your surroundings.

FIVE-STEP SELF-HOLDING[4]

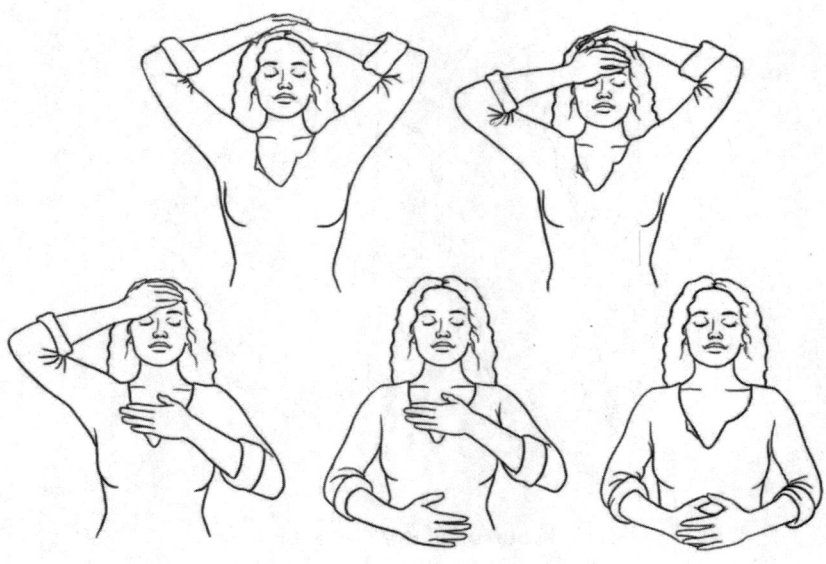

A five-step self-holding practice offers a
gentle moment of self-compassion.

From a seated shape, bring both palms to the top of your head. On
your inhale, bring your right palm over your forehead, and on your
exhale, bring your left palm over your heart. On your next inhale,
allow your right palm to rest on your belly, and as you exhale, invite
your left palm to rest over your right, bringing both palms to your
belly. Take all the time you need to gently move through these self-
compassion holds and repeat them as many times as feels supportive
to you. Feel free to offer yourself this medicine often throughout
your day.

WARRIOR I RELEASE

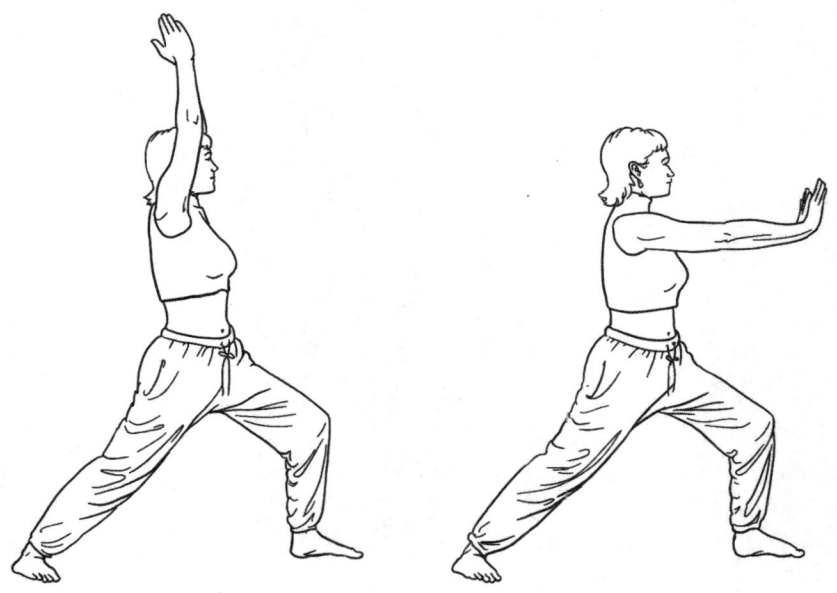

Warrior I Pose (Virabhadrasana I) is a powerful way
to shift energy and release heavy feelings.

From a standing posture, bring your right foot to the front of your
mat, slightly bending your right knee if that feels comfortable. Then
bring your left foot to the back of the mat, parallel to the edge. Rest
your hands on your hips and feel free to make any adjustments to
increase your comfort or stability.

On your inhale, extend your arms to the sky, reaching your fingertips tall and relaxing your shoulders up and back. You are welcome
to stay here for as long as it feels comfortable. On your exhale, push
your palms out and away from your body to create some space. This
is a symbolic gesture of protecting your energy and creating space to
release what feels heavy. Repeat these gestures as many times as feels
right for you and move at your own pace. Take note of any shifts you
feel mentally, emotionally, and physically as you bring this practice to
a comfortable close.

RAGDOLL RELEASE

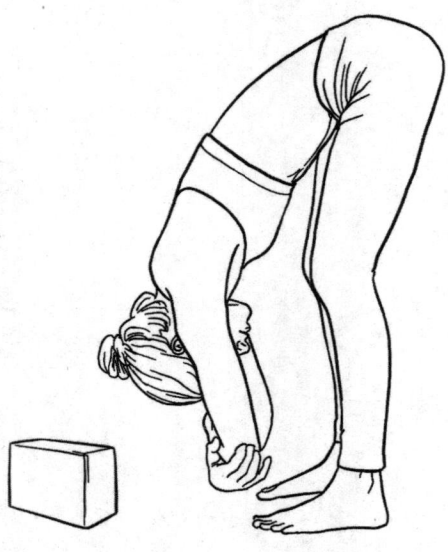

Explore Ragdoll Pose (Baddha Hasta Uttanasana) to release any tension you may be holding in your body.

Begin in a standing position and gently bring your feet hip distance apart and bring a slight bend into your knees. If it's accessible to you, gently fold forward from your hips and bend your torso into your knees. Release your fingertips toward the ground or, if it's more comfortable, place your hands onto a block, letting your head and neck hang heavy. As you bend forward, allow your body to hang freely, possibly even inviting in a gentle shaking or rocking motion to release any tension or stress you are carrying within.

Trauma-Informed Meditations for Restoration and Relief

This section includes a number of trauma-informed meditations you can drop into throughout your day for restoration and relief. To access audio recordings of these meditations, visit us.macmillan .com/ProtectYourEnergy, or perhaps you can voice-record them on your phone so you can always have them handy. If you are someone who holds space for others (e.g., yoga or meditation teacher, therapist, mental health professional, healing professional, caregiver, etc.), you can incorporate these as scripts into your work. I hope they support you. Please adapt them to your unique needs. The meditations in this section include:

- Finding Ease
- Intentional Acts of Self-Love
- An Invitation to Close Your Tabs
- Healing Is Not Linear

FINDING EASE

This meditation on finding ease is crafted to help you *soften everything*. With each inhale and exhale, explore melting a little bit deeper into your space. Do your best to really embody what it means to take in your own care, your own kindness, and your own love. Explore how you can be a little more generous, considerate, and gentle with yourself and your experience.

To begin, rest a palm on your heart and a palm on your belly, if that feels supportive and accessible to you here. Take a deep, full inhale and an audible exhale. Honor your unique pace; there is never any rush. Remember to remember yourself.

Explore bringing attention to any parts of you that need your care and take note of where you feel constriction or ease. There's no need to judge anything about your experience. Know that everything that is coming up for you is valid and welcome. If it feels okay, begin to soften a little more in places of constriction. Maybe that means softening your eyelids, softening your jaw, or relaxing your shoulders. Honor your humanity here and let the weight of what you have been carrying release from your shoulders onto the space beneath you.

In this moment, the invitation is to take up more space. If you are lying on a mat, you could rest on your back and release your arms by your sides or bring the soles of your feet to the ground and your knees together. Or perhaps you could rest on your belly and place extra support, such as a pillow or your palms, underneath your face. If you are lying on your bed, on your couch, or sitting on a cushion, you could even reach for a blanket to tend to yourself with a little more kindness and care. Continue to offer yourself the gift of your own support. As you reflect on all the ways that you hold space for others, all of the giving that you do, all of the compassion you extend daily, start to pour that back into yourself. You are worthy of extending yourself that same grace.

Now that you have taken up more space, take a deep inhale to fill up your belly and exhale at your own pace. Start to notice the energy and support of the earth beneath you and take note of how you are arriving to your practice today, honoring whatever feels close and present. Take some time here to honor your own light, allow yourself to feel held, and ponder how you can weave more moments of replenishment throughout your day amid all the output you do. Honor whatever might be unfolding for you in your practice today.

If it would feel supportive, you are welcome to connect to an intention or identify an anchor, mantra, or safe visualization you can return to if you ever come across a challenging thought in your practice. This is a pathway to support you with safely coming back home to your body and softening into your worth and your need for restoration. Perhaps spend some time reflecting on how tending to yourself in this way might ripple out into the rest of your day. How your self-care might inform your intentional choices to honor your desire for deep rest, more ease, more space, and larger margins in your day. Breathe here a little deeper, a little braver.

Continue your breath at a pace that feels supportive and nourishing. There's no need to control or constrict your breathing in any way.

Follow your own lead as you relax your shoulders once more, releasing any pressure or burdens that have come up during this practice. Inhale to draw your shoulders up and back, and exhale to relax them down your spine, letting what you are currently holding fall onto the support of the space beneath you. You were never meant to do this alone.

Be gentle with yourself as you feel your emotions and exhaustion surfacing. Start to get a little more curious and listen with compassionate awareness to your needs. Gently honor each inhale and exhale. Explore turning the volume of your heart all the way up and the volume of your thoughts all the way down.

Now bring some awareness to any sensations, moods, or energy levels you're carrying within and bringing to your practice today. There's no need to change anything about you or your experience. You are enough exactly as you are. Create space for a little more rest and a little more ease here. You might consider making a shift in the setup of your practice with an extra pillow or blanket to increase your comfort even by 5 or 10 percent. Know that you're worthy of that extra support and care.

I invite you to follow the wave of energy rising from the base of your spine and all the way to the space of your heart. Hold your intention there for a moment, if it feels right, and gently rub your palms over your heart in a soothing, circular motion. Let the strength of your body meet the power of your breath with another deep full inhale and an audible exhale.

Once again, practice softening your body from the inside out. Soften the eyelids, your brows, your jaw, and your shoulders. Reorient yourself to the sense of grounding and support from the earth beneath you, knowing that you are never alone in your experience. Allow yourself a few more moments of quiet here to reflect on your practice. To reflect on how deeply you are worthy of rest and ease. To ground yourself in the deep knowing that you have always been enough.

Take all the time you need here, and when you feel ready, invite small movements back into your body and meet me in a seated position. You're welcome to bring your palms together at the center of your heart, if that's a gesture that feels accessible to you. If not, feel free to find any other gesture that calls you. Hands at your heart, may we live our lives compassionately. Hands at your mouth, may we speak words of truth and of kindness. And hands at your third-eye center, the light in me always honors the light in you. Namaste.

INTENTIONAL ACTS OF SELF-LOVE

Take some of the radiance you pour out for others and turn it inward to shine on the neglected parts of your soul. It's time.[5]
—DR. THEMA BRYANT

This practice was crafted to help you cultivate intentional acts of self-love. In a world that constantly extracts from us, we deserve moments to pour love, care, and compassion into ourselves. May these next few moments give you the opportunity to melt into the practice of self-tending, to deeply and abundantly connect to yourself, and to honor what your heart might need.

To begin, I invite you to find a shape in your body that supports you in finding your way back home. Know that rest is deeply personal, so please choose any shape that feels supportive and nourishing in your body today. That might be sitting in a chair or on a cushion or resting on a yoga mat, a couch, or a bed. The choices you make with your body are infinitely celebrated in this space. You are the only one who gets your attention right now. I often say that showing up is the hardest part, so give yourself this space and time to prioritize your needs today.

Take a deep inhale to fill your belly with nourishing breath and exhale slowly with an open mouth. With each breath in and out, allow your body to fall into the gentleness of the space that is holding you today. On your inhale, take in your own compassion, and with each exhale, honor all parts of you here. Explore your breath in any way that feels supportive and expansive. Today you might breathe a little deeper and a little braver, acknowledging that every time you choose yourself matters.

In this moment, if it's accessible to you, rub your palms together and create a little bit of warmth. Then rest your palms over your heart space. Continue to explore your breath at your pace. I invite you to set an intention or connect to a mantra here and gently ground into your space. Know that your safety and comfort are the most important components of your practice. The hardest part is over; you have arrived and you are deeply worthy of this time.

In this space of quiet and stillness, start to explore what it looks and feels like for you to love yourself throughout this journey. If you'd like, you could gather these qualities in your mind and hold them at the space of your heart. Feel these qualities sparkling and shimmering and radiating in their fullness. Imagine just holding your self-compassion there like a beautiful glowing ball of light. If it feels safe and accessible for you, let your heart soak up those qualities.

What do the sacred parts of you need more of or less of today? Can you honor their voice? On your inhale, I invite you to take in the beauty of you and open-mouth exhale—your pace, your way.

A Few Reminders That You Deserve to Hear Often

- You deserve people in your life who honor and celebrate your choices.
- You deserve to take up space.
- You deserve your own excitement.
- You deserve your own care, your own energy, your own attention.
- You deserve to honor your progress.
- You deserve to feel full and resourced.
- You deserve larger margins in your day and space between things.
- You deserve to rest without guilt.
- You deserve to release the urgency of others.
- You deserve to schedule that appointment that you've been putting off.

- You deserve to tend to your mental health.
- You deserve to go at your pace.
- You deserve to honor your capacity.
- You deserve an abundance of grace.
- You deserve to be gentle with yourself.
- You deserve to be seen.
- You deserve your joy.
- You deserve to know that you are doing an amazing job amid it all.

As these reminders permeate your being, relax your shoulders down your spine and let the weight that you are carrying soften. Now is a good time to make any necessary shifts in your body or environment to increase your comfort. For the next part of this practice, we will move through a few gentle shapes together. If stillness feels better in your body, please honor that. This is your body, your practice, and always your choice. On your inhale, gently draw your chin up in a circular motion and then exhale to circle the chin down toward your body. Be really kind and compassionate with your movements here, so if a full neck circle feels like too much, explore a half circle instead. If you'd like, you can even invite your palms to the backs of your shoulders and give yourself a gentle self-massage. Right now where you are will always be enough.

Now bring your palms to the back of your head, extending the self-massage there. Then gently massage your temples. If it feels supportive, you could bring your energy and care to your shoulders and perhaps down your forearms, offering attention to any parts of your body that are asking for your care. It might feel nice to massage your fingers, guiding them back for a gentle stretch. Feel free to switch sides whenever you feel ready. On your next inhale, I invite you to extend your arms high to the sky, stretching your energy through your fingertips and then drawing your shoulders up and back. Hold your intention here for a moment; hold that beautiful, sparkling, shimmering light. And then exhale, bringing your palms together and resting them over your heart.

Next we will explore a heart-opening flow. On your inhale, circle your arms up and around, maybe bringing your palms together overhead. On your exhale, draw your palms and all of that loving energy to your heart. Beautiful. Repeat this movement for as many times as you would like, connecting your breath to your movement and taking in all of the energy, beauty, and intention around you.

If it feels okay, I invite you to rest a palm on your heart and a palm on your belly and draw some awareness to the concept of intentional acts of self-love. What does that mean to you? Maybe that means reminding yourself that self-care doesn't have to be something you only do at the end of your day when you've already reached that point of exhaustion and overwhelm. Maybe it's weaving moments of rest and care throughout your day. Maybe it's taking a nap, feeling the sun on your face, feeling the grass underneath your feet, or setting down all of your devices and tuning out the outside world and tuning in to you. Take another deep inhale here and exhale slowly. Spend these next few moments here in the quiet.

When you feel ready, start to invite movement back into your body in a way that feels nourishing and available in this moment. If you'd like, you can meet me in a seated position with your palms together at the center of your heart. Hands at your heart, may we live our lives compassionately. Hands at your mouth, may we speak words of truth and of kindness. And hands at your third-eye center, the light in me always honors the light in you. Namaste.

AN INVITATION TO CLOSE YOUR TABS

This is your invitation to shut down all of your devices—to close out all of your tabs, rest your mind, and find your way into any shape of rest that feels accessible to you. You could rest on your belly, curl up on your side, find a supportive shape on the couch or in your bed, or reach for a heavy blanket or an eye pillow. Perhaps this is the first moment you have had to yourself all day. Maybe you are transitioning from a really intense workweek or an overstimulating parenting day, or you're feeling the overwhelm of school or life.

Can you allow yourself to fully immerse in this moment and release the idea that your productivity determines your worth? This practice is about reclaiming and taking up space and reminding yourself that you are worthy of your own time and attention. It's about turning down the urgency of the world around you and listening to the urgency of your own care.

Maybe this is the first opportunity you've had to be still, to rest your gaze, and to actually take a deep, full breath in and out. I invite you to rub your palms together to create some warmth and then rest them over your eyes, possibly incorporating soothing circular motions to tend to any stress or tension that has accumulated throughout the day. In this moment, begin to soften everything—your shoulders, your eyelids, your brows, and your jaw. Can you let your arms fall a little bit heavier, resting them by your sides? Can you let your legs relax a bit more into the safety and support of whatever is holding you in your practice today? Allow your breath to rest here.

As you offer yourself the gift of deep rest, let this be an entry point into reclaiming your day or your evening, perhaps setting an intention around your own care. When you transition out of your meditation practice today, make a restorative plan for yourself. Breathe deeply into the sense of calm, grounding, and peace that surrounds you. Let yourself linger in the quiet for as long as you can allow. If you are doing this meditation before going to bed, perhaps you can allow yourself to doze off into this soft landing.

If you'd like to continue, I invite you to take a deep, full inhale to honor your light, and then exhale—your pace, your way. When you feel ready, you might start to invite a little bit of movement into your space to the degree that feels supportive and accessible. You could circle your ankles and wrists or wiggle your toes and fingers. You could shrug your shoulders or do some gentle neck circles. Perhaps you would like to bring your palms to the backs of your shoulders, the back of your head, your temples, or your forearms and offer yourself a self-massage. Be guided by any parts of you that need extra attention and care right now. Take your time. There's no rush.

To slowly close out your practice, you're welcome to cross your arms across your chest and take in your own care, inviting in a gentle rocking motion. You might rest your cheek on one of your palms and switch sides as it feels right. Then whenever you feel ready, bring your palms together at the center of your heart. Hands at your heart, may we live our lives compassionately. Hands at your mouth, may we speak words of truth and of kindness. And hands at your third-eye center, the light in me always honors the light in you. Namaste.

HEALING IS NOT LINEAR

This meditation was designed to remind you that the process of healing was never meant to follow a straight line and that honoring this nonlinear route allows us to approach our individual, unique, and nuanced journey with more compassion and grace. We receive so much external pressure to speed up, bounce back, and be "more resilient." Your body deserves to take as much time as it needs, and you are worthy of honoring the triggers along the way, no matter how much "work" you have done. May this meditation be a reminder that being soft with yourself is always encouraged and celebrated.

To begin, I invite you to take a deep, full inhale into the nonlinear journey that is healing. As you exhale, relax your shoulders a little bit deeper into your space. For this practice, you could keep your eyes open, find a soft gaze, or close them if that feels safe for you. You're welcome to set up your practice in any way that feels restorative—in a seated position, lying on your side or belly, or lying on your back with the soles of your feet on the mat. This is your invitation to make any necessary shifts to support your healing, rest, and care.

Today's mantra invitation is *I am present within myself. I can center myself with the ease of my breath. I feel grounded, confident, worthy, and whole. I have always been enough.* Keep this in mind as we move forward.

Explore placing your hands on your belly or giving your care to anywhere else on your body that needs your attention. Focus on taking mindful deep breaths as you scan your body, taking inventory of your needs in this moment. Know that whatever is showing up in your practice, in this space, and within your heart is welcome here. There's no need to suppress or shrink your feelings. The practice can be a bridge to support you in finding those moments of integration, healing, relief, self-worth, and joy.

Explore finding an anchor of support, perhaps feeling the energy of the earth beneath you, feeling a sense of grounding, connection, and support. Can you honor yourself and your journey and give your-self credit for how far you've come? Perhaps in this space you can invite in more compassion, more grace, and more light.

In the hard moments, remember that healing is not linear. The triggers you encounter throughout your day do not define you. You are worthy of your own support and the support of others. You are deserving of gentleness and softness, of not having to be resilient all the time.

Let the strength of your body meet the power of your breath. Feel anchored in your own wholeness, your own gentleness, your own compassion. Remind yourself often, both in your practice and in your life, that there is absolutely no rush. You deserve to take all the time you need to create space, to carve out larger margins in your day, and to dedicate time just for you. In the ebbs and flows of joy and grief, know that you are not alone in your experience. You are being held and lifted by a beautiful, courageous community that stands with you.

I invite you to continue to channel a mindful, intentional breath with this in mind. There is nothing left to do. You have already done it. You showed up for yourself and your practice today; this is the hardest part. Drop into your body, into this space you call home, and let anything that feels heavy roll off of your shoulders and onto the safety and support beneath you. Even if just for a moment within the container of this space, reconnect with today's mantra: *I am present within myself. I can center myself with the ease of my breath. I feel grounded, confident, worthy, and whole. I have always been enough.*

When you're ready, bring a little bit of movement into your space to the degree that feels right. On your inhale, explore extending your arms high; as you exhale, draw your elbows back and lift your heart to the sky for a backbend. Inhale and extend your arms high; exhale and invite your arms to rest by your sides. Perhaps you feel called to give yourself a gentle self-massage to the back of your shoulders, your forearms, the back of your head, or your temples. You choose. Your choices are beautiful. When you are settled back into your body, you are welcome to bring your palms to the center of your heart or find any other expression that's calling you here. Offer yourself more gentleness and compassion as you navigate the nonlinear routes.

As we close out this practice, I invite you to place hands at your heart, may we live our lives compassionately. Hands at your mouth, may we speak words of truth and of kindness. And hands at your third-eye center, the light in me always honors the light in you. Namaste.

Reconnecting to the Sacred Moments of Your Life

This is a sacred chapter, one I hope you can return to again and again. I wrote it intentionally to be bookmarked so when you are navigating a challenging moment, you can find your way back here to find some relief. Amid all that we experience in our lives, it can be hard to access what we might need in any given moment. I hope you can make these practices and meditations your own so they can be added to your personal healing tool kit and become second nature when you have a few minutes to tap into self-compassion, restoration, and ease. An integral part of healing your nervous system is building your capacity to cultivate more stillness in your life. Explore these practices in the in-between moments instead of scrolling on your phone or squeezing in a task, and start to track the subtle shifts they make in your daily life.

A Closing Love Note

Beloved, we have officially reached the end of this journey together, but I know in many ways it is just the beginning. If there was one thing you read that gave you a new perspective or shifted your life, I am so grateful and so deeply moved. Thank you for trusting me with your heart, your vulnerability, and your time. In moments when everything feels like too much and you forget where to begin, remember what the nervous system often needs is *less*. Begin again as many times as you need. The path will not be linear, and that is okay.

We started this journey together by exploring the gifts that slowing down, doing less, and intentionally protecting our energy can provide our nervous systems. You were reminded with courage and compassion that sometimes safety can feel like exhaustion because our bodies finally have permission to rest. We took the time and space to unpack our own narratives around the ways our bodies communicate to us through sensation and how we can lean into daily practices to help activate our parasympathetic nervous systems. We were reminded that we get to constantly redefine what success looks like for us and that growth can look like slowness for the nervous system, doing less, honoring our humanity, and processing our stress so we can work toward the cultivation of a resilient nervous system.

We gently explored the ripple impact that protecting our energy can have on all those we love, and we discussed how pouring into ourselves can allow us to show up and function in our lives with more grace. We learned that predictability and consistency can offer much-needed safety and stability for our nervous systems, that we are worthy of honoring our changing capacity and moving beyond survival to notice the moments that make us feel more awake. We ventured into the world of the window of tolerance, polyvagal theory, and finding the glimmers. And maybe, just maybe, we will finally believe that our productivity does not determine our worth.

We affirmed how exhausting it can be to always hold the default nervous system in the room, to say yes when we really want to say no, and to not check in to assess our capacity. We really started to evaluate and take note of our energy depletion, swap out draining practices for more restorative ones, reflect on the difference between having time versus having capacity, and remind ourselves of our inherent wholeness.

We spent some time getting curious about the ways our lives may feel unsustainable and how we can be more gentle and compassionate with ourselves. We reflected on our unmet needs and how we can be more intentional with prioritizing them. And we reminded ourselves of the power of cultivating our joy and finding the daily glimmers in our day through boundaries and self-inquiry. Most importantly, we embodied the reminder that boundary work is nervous system work and that quick fixes must be replaced with sustainable practices and values.

We then considered the impacts of burnout on the sensitive nervous system and discovered how building a flexible and resilient nervous system can be an anchor for so much healing to unfold. We continued to build our energy-conservation tool kit and discussed how necessary it is to tend to the undigested sensory residue that has accumulated in our bodies over time. We thought outside the box as it relates to the types of rest we need (physical, mental, emotional, creative, spiritual, sensory, and social) and explored tangible ways we can connect to deeper restoration in our lives. Finally, we closed with a number of trauma-informed healing practices including shapes of rest, compassionate meditations, and micro self-care practices we can lean into when we are looking to reduce tension and increase ease.

Intentionally tending to and nourishing our inner landscape is some of the bravest and most courageous work we will ever do.

May you always remember the power of aligning with your values, practicing compassion, honoring your boundaries, and taking up more space in your own life. As you continue on this path to protecting your energy, please stay connected and let me know how the practices in the book are landing with your heart. Join our loving community on Instagram @transcending_trauma_with_yoga and sign up for our newsletter at zabieyamasaki.com for weekly inspiration and supportive tips on your journey to reclaiming your energy and yourself. This work is deeply humbling, and holding space for you will always be my greatest honor.

Until we meet again, may you continue on your journey of protecting your most precious resource: *you.*

Acknowledgments

The journey to publishing my seventh resource in the world would not be possible without the love, belief, care, and support of so many beloveds in my life.

Thank you to my husband, Garrett, for supporting each and every endeavor and holding space for me through the intensity of fertility treatments and my writing process. We will be holding our little girl—another extension of our hearts—when this book is out in the world. I couldn't imagine life without you, and amid all we have been through, we have managed to come out the other side stronger and more connected. I love you with all my heart.

Hudson, my little love, you are currently seven years old and the kindest, most loving, magical soul. Thank you for your patience with Mommy's writing process, for setting up special stations for me to write, and for believing in the importance of Mommy's work. Everything I do is for you. I love you more than I can possibly express, sweetheart.

Leilani, you are currently growing in Mommy's belly, and we are weeks away from meeting you. Birthing this book while carrying you and meeting new versions of myself has been one of the most profound life experiences I have ever had. You've already been the greatest teacher and have taught me lessons around rest that I haven't been able to access until now. Thank you for choosing me to be your mama. You are so deeply loved and cherished.

My incredible family—Mom, Dad, Sis, Groya, Papa, and Shanni—thank you for believing in the little Zabie that dreamed of being an author one day and for supporting every endeavor of my unconventional career with so much love. Thank you for the endless childcare and support through the overwhelming moments. There is truly no one in the world like you, and there is not a day that passes that I don't realize how lucky and blessed I am that you are mine. I love you all so much.

To Almina, my beautiful sister and best friend. You've always taught me to honor my worth, and you've instilled so much in me just by being you, exactly as you are. Your unwavering love, fierce loyalty, and deep belief in me have been a constant source of strength. You have held space for me in moments of doubt and celebrated my wins like they were your own. Thank you for being my loudest cheerleader, my fiercest protector, and the kind of sister who embodies unconditional support. This book carries your energy in every page—and I am endlessly grateful to walk through life with you by my side. You are an amazing mother, daughter, sister, partner, and friend. We are all so blessed to be touched by your life.

To my amazing support system, you've all taught me that having good friends can absolutely change your life. Thank you for being there to celebrate the many ups and downs of this life, for teaching me the meaning of *unconditional*, and for always being there with a hug, a meal, and so much love. Thank you for being so good for my nervous system. I am so blessed to be touched by your light.

To my boo/bestie Jules, how you manage all that you do as a surgeon, a mother, and a wife with so much grace and still show up for me in all of the ways astounds me. You are such a special soul, and I will always be here to remind you of your light. Thank you for holding me through life's most trying moments and never giving up on the hope of all we have imagined and dreamed in our lives. I think of the college version of us; twenty-plus years later, I can't believe all the ways we have grown up together. Your friendship is the greatest gift to my heart. I could never manage this lifetime without you.

To my soul sister/bestie Sahar, thank you for being you. You've healed my heart in so many ways through your endless support and friendship. You've been the biggest cheerleader of my work. You always know just what to say. I am constantly in awe of you, the various identities you hold, and how you manage to show up for every person who is so blessed to be touched by your life. Cheers to the many life milestones we will continue to share together. May you always honor your light and know how loved and cherished you are. I truly can't imagine my life without you.

To Sabrina, you have fundamentally changed my business and my life. I am in awe of you constantly, and I hope you see your own light. Thank you for making my life lighter and more manageable and for always anticipating my needs and preventing my breakdowns! You are passionate, loving, and incredible at everything you do. You are a one-of-a-kind human and I am so lucky to know you. Transcending Trauma through Yoga would not be what it is today without you.

To my one-of-a-kind literary agent Laura Lee at Present Perfect Literary, your fierce advocacy and belief in my work has been so moving to witness. You are such a gem, and you're doing life-changing work. Thank you from the bottom of my heart for all you have done to bring my work to light and for being such a joy and pleasure.

To my amazing publishing team at Sounds True (now a part of St. Martin's Essentials)—Diana, Sarah, Jade, and Lyric—thank you for pouring the time, care, and love you have into this book; for believing in it and breathing so much life, intention, and radiance into it; and for simply being incredible humans to work with.

Additional Resources

Resource 1: Nervous System Care Checklist

Nervous system health is a foundational practice to being human in these times.

Because this book is focused on protecting your energy, I wanted this to be one of the first support resources you become familiar with. When our nervous systems experience dysregulation, it can be challenging to identify what, exactly, might help. One of the hardest parts of dysregulation is that it sweeps us *out* of the moment and away from rational thinking, so any sort of decision—even deciding which tool might help us get resourced—becomes difficult. The invitations on this care plan are meant to be an accessible, tangible, supportive, and comforting tool for those moments of overwhelm, exhaustion, and crisis.

My hope is that having a reference like this alleviates some of the pressure you might have inadvertently put on yourself. Whether you're barely holding it together, looking for ways to practice preventative self-care, or feeling the ongoing grief of navigating these times, I hope there is something here you can draw from. I hope it holds you in all the ways you are deserving. Be gentle with yourself.

For a downloadable version of this worksheet, visit us.macmillan.com/ProtectYourEnergy or use this QR code.

PHYSICAL

- Take a few moments to stretch in bed.
- Move my body simply because it brings me joy.
- Schedule a walking meeting.
- Lie down and rest my eyes for ten minutes.
- Take a warm bath.
- Practice gentleness with my experience and tend to my basic needs.
- Connect with practices that activate my parasympathetic nervous system.
- Take a power nap.
- Drink a glass of water.
- Eat a nourishing meal.
- Be patient and compassionate with myself when resting is hard.

EMBODIMENT PRACTICES TO EXPLORE

- Five-step compassion hold
- Supported Child's Pose (Balasana)
- Compassionate face cradle
- Heart and ear soothing
- Sun meditation to thaw grief
- Self-massage
- Butterfly hug

MENTAL

- Decline a request.
- Practice building in buffers or margins between meetings.
- Block off and protect time on my calendar.
- Cancel or reschedule something.
- Communicate a boundary that is on my heart.
- Let someone else volunteer.
- Give myself permission to release something from today's list.
- Read something that sparks inspiration and ease.

PHRASES TO EASE YOUR NERVOUS SYSTEM

- "Give yourself grace."
- "Take your time. You don't have to rush."
- "Be gentle with yourself."
- "You don't have to overextend yourself to be worthy."
- "It's okay to release the pressure of being resilient all the time. Resilience can also look like rest."
- "Ease is available to me."

EMOTIONAL

- Make a plan to prioritize and communicate my needs and get them met.
- Affirm my feelings just as they are.
- Ask for help.
- Cry, process, release.
- Be gentle with myself.
- Schedule a mental health day.
- Portion my time and honor my capacity and energy.
- Offer myself the gift of my own compassion.

SPIRITUAL

- Do meditative practices in nature.
- Do one thing to replenish my spirit.
- Practice sensory self-care.
- Practice releasing the urgency.
- Practice compassion and grace with everything I am holding.
- Watch the sunset, find presence, connect to joy from an embodied place.
- Choose to do less even if more feels like an option.
- Practice an energy protection meditation.

ADD YOUR OWN

-
-
-
-
-

Resource 2: Assessing Your Energy Worksheet

This worksheet provides a way for you to steward your energy throughout the day. Feel welcome to make this your own, fill out only what you feel called to, and allow it to be a supportive tool to help you be more intentional with honoring your energy and capacity each day.

For a downloadable version of this worksheet, visit us.macmillan .com/ProtectYourEnergy.

Date:

MORNING

Energy check-in (free-flow description of your current energy; e.g., full, depleted, grounded, frenetic):

Time:

What type of day is ahead, beloved?:

Anchoring and grounding intention:

- Peace
- Boundaries
- Compassion
- Energy
- Ease
- Rest
- Connection
- Mindfulness
- Other:

My rest affirmation and reminder (e.g., I am worthy of resting before I am exhausted):

AFTERNOON

Energy check-in (free-flow description of your current energy; e.g., full, depleted, grounded, frenetic):

Time:

Plans for tending to your nervous system:
Are there one or two things from this list you can connect to in this moment?

- Hydrate.
- Stretch in bed.
- Walk in nature.
- Schedule appointment that has been pushed off.
- Engage in movement/meditation.
- Delegate tasks.
- Release the urgency.
- Make a plan to prioritize and communicate my needs and then get them met.
- Decline someone's request.
- Take a power nap.
- Unplug/honor sensory self-care.
- Block off and protect time on my calendar.
- Do one thing to replenish my spirit.
- Tend to my basic needs.
- Ask for help.
- Cancel or reschedule something.
- Communicate a boundary.
- Find the glimmers.
- Eat a nourishing meal.
- Resist the urge to "power through."
- Connect with community that supports my mental health and nervous system.
- Lie down and do nothing.
- Read something that sparks inspiration and ease.

- Give myself permission to release a task from today's list.
- Watch the sunset.
- Let someone else take the lead.
- Journal.
- Affirm my feelings just as they are.
- Practice an embodied check-in before taking on additional commitments.
- Take my full lunch break not in front of a screen.
- Choose to do less, even if more is an option.
- My ideas:

EVENING

Energy check-in (free-flow description of your current energy; e.g., full, depleted, grounded, frenetic):

Time:

Sunshine and cloud of the day (e.g., What went well today? Where did I struggle?):

Ways I practiced compassion with my experience:

Other reflections:

Intentions to guide tomorrow:

Resource 3: Types of Rest Worksheet

This worksheet is a quick tool you can use to parse out what kind of rest your body may be craving and provide examples of rest that could offer some relief. Feel free to pick what works for you, and I encourage you to implement these forms of rest into your daily life. These preventative self-care ideas are inspired by Dr. Saundra Dalton-Smith's "Seven Types of Rest" framework. For a downloadable version of this worksheet, visit us.macmillan.com/ProtectYourEnergy.

PHYSICAL REST

- Passive physical rest: sleeping, napping, restorative Yoga Nidra, sleep meditation/podcast, acupuncture, massage, sound healing class
- Active physical rest: yoga, stretching, reading on the couch with a cozy blanket, anything that allows you to tend to your body with care and love
- Prioritizing doctors' appointments for yourself
- Tending to yourself before a busy time instead of waiting until you have reached exhaustion
- Practicing doing daily tasks, such as eating or running errands, slowly instead of completing them "real quick"
- Managing your energy instead of your time

EMOTIONAL REST

- Creating intentional time for yourself, such as therapy, hiking, or cuddling
- Not giving all of yourself away during the day
- Postponing or canceling events on your calendar during a hard week
- Delegating tasks rather than taking the lead

MENTAL REST

- Taking a break from holding the default nervous system in the room
- Allowing yourself to not carry it all
- Creating space between tasks in your day
- Closing your tabs
- Journaling and indulging in stillness
- Doing nothing
- Lowering expectations for yourself

CREATIVE REST

- Immersing yourself in environments that awaken your sense of awe, wonder, and passion
- Finding the glimmers and micro-moments of joy in your day
- Making time for a hobby you love (pottery, karaoke, roller-skating)
- Putting on your favorite outfit

SPIRITUAL REST

- Connecting to a deep sense of belonging, love, community, acceptance, and purpose
- Engaging in a restorative daily ritual
- Joining a faith-based community and/or prayer circle
- Spending time in nature
- Meditating or doing some contemplative practices
- Listening to a restorative or spiritual playlist
- Setting boundaries with people who drain you

SENSORY REST

- Intentionally unplugging from technology
- Engaging in repetition, ritual, and routine for your senses

- Building in mindful transition time (e.g., washing your face, meditating, sitting in silence, going for a walk, cuddling a pet)
- Drinking a comforting beverage
- Looking out the window to daydream
- Wearing soft, comfortable clothes
- Taking breaks from absorbing the news or other overstimulating information

SOCIAL REST

- Sorting out the relationships that revive you versus the relationships that exhaust you
- Reflecting on how each person, space, etc., impacts your mind, body, and spirit
- Leaving texts unread until you have more time and energy to respond
- Declining social requests when you are low on capacity
- Taking a social media break
- Spending time with people who fill your cup

Notes

Epigraphs

Epigraph 1: Thaís Sky (@IamThaisSky), X, August 22, 2021, x.com/IamThaisSky/status/1429623666527014918.

Epigraph 2: Hannah Rosenberg, "Until I Thought of Myself as the Sea," *HannahRoWrites*, July 18, 2022, hannahrowrites.substack.com/p/until-i-thought-of-myself-as-the.

Introduction

1   Nakeia Homer (@NakeiaHomer), X, June 29, 2022, x.com/NakeiaHomer/status/1542324202069495808.
2   Angela Y. Davis, *Women, Culture & Politics* (Vintage, 2011).
3   Dr. Thema Bryant (@drthema), X, July 1, 2021, x.com/drthema/status/1410807926059507712?lang=en.
4   Nicola Jane Hobbs, *The Relaxed Woman: Reclaim Rest and Live an Empowered, Joy-Filled Life* (Penguin Group, 2025).
5   Kathryn Nicolai, host, *Nothing Much Happens*, season 14, episode 26, "Retreat (Encore)," August 29, 2024, nothingmuchhappens.com/stories/the-retreat-encore.
6   Northwestern Medicine Staff, "Health Benefits of Having a Routine," Northwestern Medicine, December 14, 2022, nm.org/healthbeat/healthy-tips/health-benefits-of-having-a-routine.

Chapter 1: Your Nervous System Is Your Friend and Teacher

1   Abby Rawlinson (@therapywithabby), Instagram, December 13, 2024, instagram.com/p/DDgvN05o1_o/.
2   Deb Dana, *Polyvagal Exercises for Safety and Connection: 50 Client-Centered Practices* (W. W. Norton, 2020).
3   MedicTests, *Adrenergics/Anti-Adrenergics and Cholinergics/Anti-Cholinergics | MedicTests.* (n.d.), medictests.com/units/adrenergics-anti-adrenergics-and-cholinergics-anti-cholinergics#:~:text=PARASYMPATHETIC%20NERVOUS%20SYSTEM%20(the%20Cholinergic,neurotransmitter%3A%20ACETYLCHOLINE%20(ACh).
4   Jennifer Mann and Karden Rabin, *The Secret Language of the Body: Regulate Your Nervous System, Heal Your Body, Free Your Mind* (HarperCollins UK, 2024).
5   Jim Kwik (@jimkwik), X, October 17, 2022, x.com/jimkwik/status/1582072454528147456?lang=en.
6   We the Urban (@wetheurban), Instagram, n.d., instagram.com/wetheurban/.
7   Arielle Schwartz, *Therapeutic Yoga for Trauma Recovery: Applying the Principles of Polyvagal Theory for Self-Discovery, Embodied Healing, and Meaningful Change* (PESI Publishing, 2022).
8   Meg Josephson (@megjosephson), Instagram, November 5, 2023, instagram.com/p/CzRhAOGvKs1/.
9   Dana, *Polyvagal Exercises for Safety and Connection.*
10 Schwartz, *Therapeutic Yoga for Trauma Recovery.*
11 Abby Rawlinson, *Reclaiming You: Your Therapy Toolkit for Life's Twists and Turns* (Random House, 2024).
12 Thaís Sky (@IamThaisSky), Instagram, n.d., instagram.com/iamthaissky/.
13 Brianna Pastor, *Good Grief* (Hachette UK, 2024).
14 Tricia Hersey, *Rest Is Resistance: A Manifesto* (Hachette UK, 2022).

15　Kimani Fambro (@kimanifambro), Instagram, n.d., instagram.com/kimanifambro/?hl=en.

16　Sophie Cliff, *Choose Joy: Relieve Burnout, Focus on Your Happiness, and Infuse More Joy into Your Everyday Life* (Blue Star Press, 2022).

17　Cliff, *Choose Joy.*

18　Dana, *Polyvagal Exercises for Safety and Connection.*

19　Helen Marie, *Choose You: Gentle Words to Help You Heal and Grow* (Random House, 2024).

Chapter 2: How to Assess and Protect Your Energy

1　Joél Leon (@iamjoelleon), Instagram, n.d., instagram.com/iamjoelleon/.

2　Amber Lyon (@modernmind___), Instagram, December 2, 2024, instagram.com/modernmind___/p/DDFT9vyp7m_/.

3　Wildfaith (@wildfaithpoetry), Instagram, n.d., instagram.com/wildfaithpoetry/.

4　Jenn Granneman and Andre Sólo, *Sensitive: The Hidden Power of the Highly Sensitive Person in a Loud, Fast, Too-Much World* (National Geographic Books, 2023).

5　Jo Buick (@jo.buick), Instagram, n.d., instagram.com/jo.buick/.

6　Nicola Jane Hobbs, *The Relaxed Woman: Reclaim Rest and Live an Empowered, Joy-Filled Life* (G. P. Putnam's Sons, 2025).

7　Ximena Vengoechea, *Rest Easy: Discover Calm and Abundance through the Radical Power of Rest* (Chronicle Books, 2023).

8　Katherine Morgan Schafler, *The Perfectionist's Guide to Losing Control* (Hachette UK, 2023).

9　Becky Kennedy, *Good Inside: A Practical Guide to Becoming the Parent You Want to Be* (HarperCollins UK, 2022).

10　James Clear, *Atomic Habits: An Easy and Proven Way to Build Good Habits and Break Bad Ones* (Random House, 2018).

Chapter 3: You Can't—and Shouldn't—Do It All

1 Jonathan Louis Dent (@jonathanldent), Instagram, n.d., instagram.com/jonathanldent/.
2 Alex Elle (@alex_elle), Instagram, n.d., instagram.com/alex_elle/.
3 Madeleine Dore, *I Didn't Do the Thing Today: On Letting Go of Productivity Guilt* (Allen & Unwin, 2022).
4 Tracee Stanley, host, *Radiant Rest*, podcast, bonus episode, "Empowering Children to Thrive with Crystal McCreary," March 29, 2022, radiantrest.com/bonus-episode-empowering-children-to-thrive-with-crystal-mccreary/.
5 Jennifer Cohen Harper (@jennifercohenharper), Instagram, January 1, 2022, instagram.com/p/CYMd0Ivr6aV/?img_index=1.
6 Pooja Lakshmin, *Real Self-Care: A Transformative Program for Redefining Wellness (Crystals, Cleanses, and Bubble Baths Not Included)* (National Geographic Books, 2023).
7 Tim Ferriss, host, *The Tim Ferriss Show*, shorts, "'Marriage Is Never 50/50'—Brené Brown," June 5, 2023, youtube.com/watch?v=yfL4RTuC9Bk.
8 Ashley Neese, host, *The Deeper Call*, "Embodying Our Inherent Value with Zabie Yamasaki," October 4, 2023, Spotify, open.spotify.com/episode/1RhJqaTpESwnorm45R27Nu?si=dd49cb72d3c644ec&nd=1&dlsi=e206d9453cd24d86.

Chapter 4: Restoring the Nervous System Through Embodied Boundaries

1 Ronne Brown, posted by Navucko (@navucko), Instagram, August 29, 2024, instagram.com/navucko/p/C_QU8r1smIp/.
2 Helen Marie, *Choose You: Gentle Words to Help You Heal and Grow* (Random House, 2024), 174.
3 Marie, *Choose You*, 174.

4   Ashley Neese, *Permission to Rest: Revolutionary Practices for Healing, Empowerment, and Collective Care* (Ten Speed Press, 2023), 25.

5   Nedra Glover Tawwab, *Set Boundaries, Find Peace: A Guide to Reclaiming Yourself* (Hachette UK, 2021).

6   Tawwab, *Set Boundaries, Find Peace.*

7   Becky Kennedy, *Good Inside: A Practical Guide to Becoming the Parent You Want to Be* (HarperCollins UK, 2022).

8   Prentis Hemphill (@prentishemphill), Instagram, April 5, 2021, instagram.com/prentishemphill/p/CNSzFO1A21C/.

Chapter 5: A Mind, Body, and Spirit Approach to Unwinding from Burnout

1   Brianna Pastor, *Good Grief* (Hachette UK, 2024).

2   Tara Haelle, "Your 'Surge Capacity' Is Depleted—It's Why You Feel Awful," *Elemental*, August 17, 2020, sog.unc.edu/sites /default/files/course_materials/Your%20Surge%20Capacity %20is%20Depleted.pdf.

3   Emily Nagoski and Amelia Nagoski, *Burnout: The Secret to Unlocking the Stress Cycle* (Random House, 2019).

4   Amelia Nagoski and Emily Nagoski, "What Is the Stress Cycle and How Can You Complete It?" posted April 8, 2019, by Ebury Reads, youtube.com/watch?v=CyppUSV1FN0.

5   Jennifer Mann and Karden Rabin, *The Secret Language of the Body: Regulate Your Nervous System, Heal Your Body, Free Your Mind* (HarperCollins UK, 2024).

6   Pooja Lakshmin, *Real Self-Care: A Transformative Program for Redefining Wellness (Crystals, Cleanses, and Bubble Baths Not Included)* (National Geographic Books, 2023).

7   Cleopatra (@amandaperera), X, October 17, 2022, x.com /amandaperera/status/1582034238097924096.

8   Nicole Steward, *Radical Self-Care for Helpers, Healers, and Changemakers* (W. W. Norton, 2025).

9   Shena J. Young, *Body Rites: A Holistic Healing and Embodiment Workbook for Black Survivors of Sexual Trauma* (W. W. Norton, 2023).

10 Bo Forbes, *Yoga for Emotional Balance: Simple Practices to Help Relieve Anxiety and Depression* (Shambhala Publications, 2011).

11 Eleanor Criswell, Amy Wheeler, and Mary Partlow Lauttamus, "Yoga Therapy Research, Individualized Yoga Therapy and Call It Yoga Therapy," *International Journal of Yoga Therapy* 24, no. 1 (2024): 2329, doi.org/10.17761/ijyt.24.1 .a472jr148535634j.

12 Edutopia (@edutopia), Instagram, November 11, 2020, instagram.com/edutopia/p/CHdF0tNFvwJ/.

13 Dorcas Cheng-Tozun, *Social Justice for the Sensitive Soul: How to Change the World in Quiet Ways* (Broadleaf Books, 2023), 13.

14 Linnea Passaler, *Heal Your Nervous System: The 5-Stage Plan to Reverse Nervous System Dysregulation* (Fair Winds Press, 2024).

Chapter 6: The Intentional Practice of Rest

1   Manassaline (@sa.liine), Instagram, November 1, 2024, instagram.com/p/DB1j-jcSTye/.

2   L. E. Bowman (@l.e.bowman.poetry), Instagram, November 9, 2024, instagram.com/p/DCJ9jexO7IW/.

3   Tracee Stanley, *Radiant Rest: Yoga Nidra for Deep Relaxation and Awakened Clarity* (Shambhala Publications, 2021).

4   Ximena Vengoechea, *Rest Easy: Discover Calm and Abundance through the Radical Power of Rest* (Chronicle Books, 2023).

5   Tricia Hersey, *Rest Is Resistance: A Manifesto* (Hachette UK, 2022).

6   Rainesford Stauffer, *All the Gold Stars: Reimagining Ambition and the Ways We Strive* (Hachette UK, 2023).

7   Alexis Florentina (@lexyflorentina), Instagram, n.d., instagram.com/lexyflorentina/.

8   Saundra Dalton-Smith, "The Real Reason Why We Are Tired and What to Do about It," TEDxAtlanta, March 2019,

ted.com/talks/saundra_dalton_smith_the_real_reason_why
_we_are_tired_and_what_to_do_about_it.

9 Zahabiyah Yamasaki, *Trauma-Informed Yoga Flip Chart: A Teaching Tool for Healing Professionals* (W. W. Norton, 2024).

Chapter 7: Micro Self-Care Practices and Trauma-Informed Meditations to Protect Your Energy

1 Dr. Thema Bryant (@drthema), X, December 5, 2023, x.com /drthema/status/1732224982665810392.

2 Madison Abdallah (@radiantsomatics), Instagram, n.d., instagram.com/radiantsomatics/.

3 Shena J. Young, *Body Rites: A Holistic Healing and Embodiment Workbook for Black Survivors of Sexual Trauma* (W. W. Norton, 2023).

4 Peter Levine, *Healing Trauma: A Pioneering Program for Restoring the Wisdom of Your Body* (Sounds True, 2008).

5 Dr. Thema Bryant (@drthema), X, August 30, 2020, x.com /drthema/status/1300279716910260224.

About the Author

Zabie Yamasaki (she/her), MEd, RYT, is the founder of Transcending Trauma through Yoga, which is an organization that offers trauma-informed yoga to survivors, consultations to universities and trauma agencies, and training for healing professionals. Zabie is widely recognized for her intentionality, soulful activism, and passionate dedication to her field. She has trained thousands of healing professionals, yoga instructors, and mental health practitioners in her signature trauma-informed yoga certification both in person and online. She is a trauma-informed yoga instructor, resilience and well-being educator, and a sought-after consultant and keynote speaker. Her program and curriculum is now being implemented at more than fifty college campuses and trauma agencies across the country including the University of California (UC) system, Stanford, Yale, University of Southern California, University of Notre Dame, and Johns Hopkins University. Her work has been highlighted on CNN, NBC, KTLA 5, and HuffPost.

Zabie received her undergraduate degree in psychology and social behavior and education at University of California, Irvine, and her graduate degree in higher education administration and student affairs at the George Washington University. She is the author of several publications including: *Trauma-Informed Yoga for Survivors of Sexual Assault: Practices for Healing and Teaching with Compassion*; *Trauma-Informed Yoga Affirmation Card Deck*; *Trauma-Informed Yoga Flip Chart: A Teaching Tool for Healing Professionals*; *Your Joy Is Beautiful: The Magic of Remembering That You Are Enough,*

Just As You Are; and *H Is for Healing Card Deck: 52 Everyday Practices to Strengthen Children's Emotional, Physical, and Mental Well-Being.*

You can learn more about her work, trainings, and speaking engagements at zabieyamasaki.com or on Instagram @transcending_trauma_with_yoga.

About Sounds True Books

Sounds True was founded in 1985 by Tami Simon with a clear man-date: to disseminate spiritual wisdom. Since starting out as a project with one woman and her tape recorder, Sounds True has grown into a mission-driven learning and media company, partnering with many of the leading wisdom teachers and visionaries of our time.

Every Sounds True Book is designed to not only provide infor-mation to a reader but to also to embody the quality of a wisdom transmission, unlocking our greatest capacities to love, serve, and uplift others.

Sounds True Books are part of St. Martin's Essentials, an imprint of Macmillan Publishers.